TO COMMAND IS TO SERVE

That's A True Pharma First-Line Leader

Foreword by

VIVEK HATTANGADI

Rajat Saha

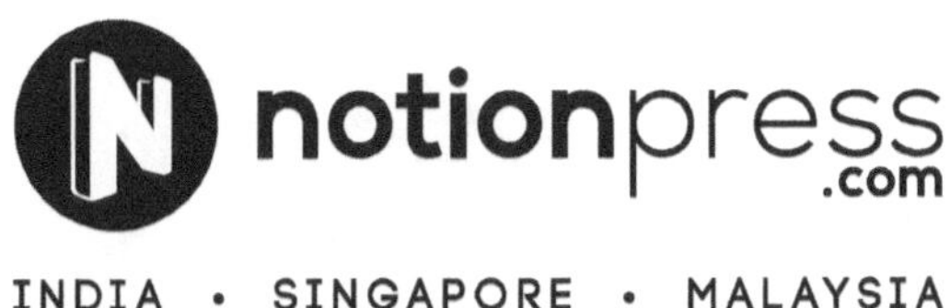

INDIA • SINGAPORE • MALAYSIA

ISBN 978-1-68466-715-4

CONTENTS

FOREWORD

Tom Peters says: "While first-line managers are considered to be of great importance, in my experience few companies truly obsess on every aspect of their care and feeding. In fact, my observations suggest that such things as First-line Leader training regimes are often of questionable quality. This is a strategic mistake – More important, a lost strategic opportunity."

Sadly, Pharma India has not learnt that investment on First-line leader's continuous learning and development is going to pay massive dividends in the long-term period. Ultimately we have a large army of super-duper medical representatives posing as First-line leaders and delivering mediocre results.

Who is to be blamed? The organization or the First-line leader himself? I won't answer this question but here is an opportunity for all those First-line leaders who want to be the self-learners – irrespective of the priorities of their organization!

This wonderful book **"TO COMMAND IS TO SERVE – THAT'S A TRUE PHARMA FIRST-LINE LEADER"** is for those who are keen to develop themselves.

"TO COMMAND IS TO SERVE – THAT'S A TRUE PHARMA FIRST-LINE LEADER" is a comprehensive primer not just for those currently in the First-line leadership cadre but is also for those medical representatives who want to make progress in their careers. One thing which First-line leaders, especially the newly promoted must learn is that their role, by stretch assignment is even more demanding than anticipated. They have to learn that the skills and the mindset required for success as a manager is starkly different – and that there is a gap between their current capabilities and what is expected from them to succeed as a First-line leader.

As medical representatives their success depended primarily on their skills to generate prescriptions. Now is the time to develop their people so that medical representatives are able to generate prescriptions. The First-line leader is no more a prescription generator. And a novice First-line leader can't afford to learn this by trial and error.

This book vividly brings about how to cope up with the new job as a First-line leader. Importantly, First-line leader will also learn how to manage as leaders, even if in adverse conditions, such as under pressure.

The book covers all essential topics such as emotional wellness and intelligence, body language, leadership, motivation, managing time, dealing with superiors, and much more. The book is written in an inviting style, with relevant illustrations and case studies. I recommend this book to all First-line leaders!

Vivek Hattangadi

THANKS GIVING

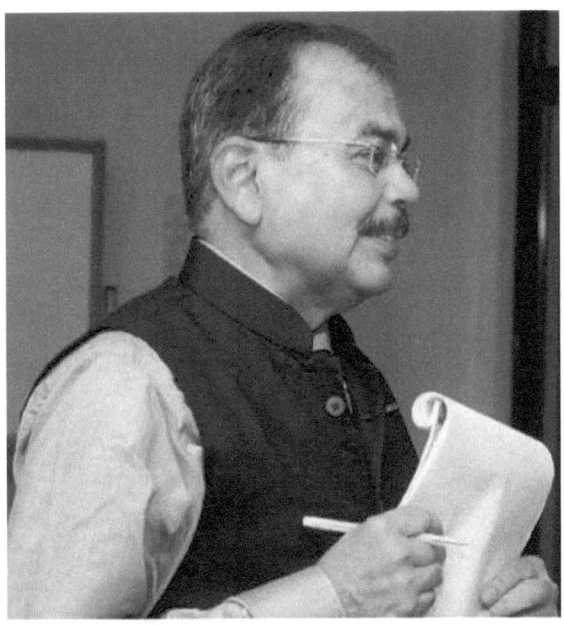

Just like my previous book, *You Can Be A Medical Representative,* once again for this book, I will always remain thankful to my mentor Mr. Vivek Hattangadi, Chief Mentor, "The Enablers" who instigated my thought processes to write down my thoughts.

ACKNOWLEDGEMENT

I am very grateful to all who gave valuable insights into preparing *To Command Is To Serve.* The basic outline and concise curriculum they helped me was easy to understand and use. Without their valuable guidance, this book would not have been a reality. This book is an essence of my personal experience and the learning and training provided to me by the organizations I worked with.

I would like to thank Mr. Dhritiman Chatterjee, Kolkata, Dr. Bikash Rai Das, Guwahati for their valuable guidance and inspiration.

Finally, I would like to acknowledge the support of Suparna, my wife and Raaina, my daughter. Without their support, it would not have been possible for me to complete this book.

Rajat Saha

INTRODUCTION

Over the last couple of decades the world has been experiencing immense change and the business environment has grown dramatically more intense. Competitions are now more acute than ever before. *'Management has been defined as getting results through others.'* Today, management simply isn't sufficient anymore. The nature of managerial work is changing because people today are no longer commanded or bossed. People have become less negotiable. No longer can managers simply issue orders and expect them to be thoughtlessly obeyed. The industry is too unpredictable, too volatile for such a management approach.

What's needed now is LEADER. You cannot do it by directive anymore. It has to be by influence. A leader is a person who goes in the front, leads the way by his/her actions; people follow. A leader ensures that the team members give their best willingly. In today's world, people get attracted to leadership. They follow a good leader and try to act like them.

Leading people is a complex task as it demands effective communication, interpersonal awareness, commitment, motivation and the ability to influence. In current scenario, organisations are desperate need of effective leaders capable of producing results. It is the leader who can transform the organisation.

Leadership is the ability of a person to influence, motivate and enable others to contribute towards the effectiveness and success of the organisation. Leadership is a fascinating aspect gaining increasing importance in business organisations. It is the process of influencing people to perform assigned tasks willingly, efficiently and competently.

Leadership is an important function of management which helps to maximise efficiency and to achieve organisational goals. Leadership and management are closely linked functions. Both the functions are complementary to each other. Leadership and management operate hand in hand. To be an effective manager, the manager needs leadership skills, and an effective leader depends on the management skills for achieving the goals and objectives. Perhaps, leadership is an essential part and an important component of effective management.

The pharmaceutical industry across the globe is changing and the competition is becoming aggressive day by day. Pharmaceutical industry in India is among the fastest growing areas producing a large number of jobs. The number of companies as well as the number of sales people has increased considerably. ***The post of a First-Line Manager is the most important position because they form the backbone of the pharmaceutical industry.*** Technically it is a first-line manager's role also called Area Manager, Area Business Manager or District Manager in various organisations. ***First-line managers must have traits of a leader. They must possess leadership qualities.*** With leadership qualities the first-line manager can build and sustain competitive advantage. First-line leadership determines excellent organisational performance.

The pharma first-line leader is usually responsible for handling a particular territory with few medical representatives. They are at the very first level of management. The first-line leadership is about leading a team of medical representatives to produce a set of business outcomes. They are the key to high performance because they spend more time with medical representatives who actually generate the revenue for the organisation. First-line leaders can lead their teams by motivating them in a positive way, that they should achieve their objectives every month with the help of the company's strategy which should be 100% implemented in the field.

A Pharma first-line leader is a professional whose nature of work is challenging and highly competitive. Perhaps, today's competitive environment has put pressure on them as they have direct exposure to the challenges faced by the industry. The first-line position is the most important because a Pharmaceutical organisation is solid or weak that relies upon first-line leaders. They are the key to organisational performance and business results and they need to be provided with the right knowledge and skills set to do the job.

'To Command Is To Serve – That's A True Pharma First-Line Leader' is a simple practical guide for those who is about to take up the position of a first-line manager in an organisation and this book will be equally useful for the existing first-line managers who wish to improve their leadership skills. If you are at first-line position, this book will give you a complete framework for becoming an effective leader. However, the principles of leadership are same in any field of work.

'Leadership, like swimming, cannot be learned by reading about it.' However, you can learn about first-line leadership only when you make a conscious effort to relate the points to your real life experience.

I don't consider myself as expert on the subjects; I feel confident that my experience in the leadership position can help my readers a lot. After poring through many books and articles written by many experts and putting to practice their advice, I decided to give expression to all my experience in the shape of a book.

I would consider my efforts a success if this book can be of some help to Pharma First-Line Leaders. All suggestions for improvement are cordially welcome.

Rajat Saha

CHAPTER 1

PHARMA FIRST-LINE LEADER

WHO IS A LEADER?

> ***'If your action inspire others to dream more, learn more, do more and become more, then you are a Leader'***
>
> ***– John Quincy Adams***

A leader is someone who influences a group of people towards the achievement of a goal. The term 'leader' refers to anyone, in any field, who significantly influences others. The leader is a person who leads and the objective of a leader is to get his/her team from where they are to where they have never been. A leader can enable the team members to accomplish their potential by constantly challenging them to do more by stretching them and helping them get through their restrictions and start believing in their abilities. In fact, leaders act as a catalyst for enhancing the effectiveness of the team members.

Leadership is an essential factor for making an organisation successful. The word 'leadership' refers to the ability to lead and is defined simply as *displaying the skills of a leader.* It is a process of directing and influencing a group of people. Leadership is all about focused action towards commendable reason. Leadership is a perspective; it's about vision, spirit and character and getting different individuals to work together as a team. Leadership is about having unshakeable confidence in your vision and persistent trust in your power to make positive change happen.

The idea about leadership has been changed. In the current scenario, people can no longer be commanded or bossed about in the same way as before. Leadership today is about working extraordinarily well with and through others. You need to remove the bureaucratic roadblocks as much as possible and manage horizontally.

'Leadership cannot really be taught; it can only be learned'
– Harold Geneen

'The quality of leadership determines the success or failure of an organisation.' In a competitive business environment, effective leadership is an essential requirement in order to achieve organisational goals. Leadership has become the single most important master skill for growth of an organisation.

Leadership is interesting and complex; however organisation can give you position and authority but does not make you a leader. Becoming a leader doesn't happen overnight, and is one of the hardest things to get right. Leadership development is a lifetime journey; it's something you need to continuously work at. Leadership happens when a person allows you to influence his or her lives. It's only when your influence causes him or her to work towards a shared vision that you become a leader.

'Management is a position that is gained; Leadership a status that is earned'

LEADERSHIP STARTS WITH LEADING ONESELF

The foundation of leadership is self-leadership. Before developing leadership skills, it is necessary that one must take complete control over oneself. If you wish to lead, invest at least 50% of your time in leading yourself. You have to be the master of your own life. *'Leadership in your world begins with leadership with your life.'* If you can't lead yourself then it will be troublesome for you to lead others. Continuous improvement, on-going personal and professional development can help you be ever better in your role as a leader.

'Great organisations begin with great Leaders. If you have the desire and willpower you can become an effective leader. Great leaders develop through a never-ending process of self-study, education, training and experience.' The great leaders recognise that leadership is a craft, not a gift. They constantly work to refine their art.

> ***'Leaders aren't born, they are made. And they are made just like anything else, through hard work. And that's the price we'll have to pay to achieve that goal, or any goal.'***
>
> ***– Vince Lombardi***

ANYONE CAN BE A LEADER

'Leadership is learned and everyone has the potential to be a leader'

We are born with equal potential. Every one of us has the potential to be a leader every day. Anyone who is willing to make the effort can become a leader. Leadership is not just about the head of the organisation or the captain of the team. It's about each one of us. Anyone can be a leader. *'Leadership is not just by rank or designation; it is by action.'* Robin Sharma, in his book has pointed out that, you don't have to have a title to be a leader. He states that we all must step up to the mark and be a leader in our own field, even if we work in a team or are self-employed. This can be illustrated by following example:

"In Mumbai terror attack of November 26, 2008, Tukaram Omble, an assistant police sub inspector, took a leadership position. He marched ahead, taking bullets on his chest, but caught Ajmal kasab alive. Omble proved his leadership, irrespective of his designation. As the saying goes, 'when the going gets tough, the tough get going.' This is initiative and this is Leadership."

As a first-line leader your actions will say much more to your medical representatives, about your values and your leadership skills than your words ever can. When you think about leadership, think about actions.

> ***'It is the action, not the words which determines Leadership'***

Leadership is simply a way of thinking, or 'mindset.' To become a leader, you need to change your mindset. Our thoughts guide us towards the actions we take. Leadership is about having the entrepreneur mindset, and anyone can develop this mindset. Entrepreneurial comes from a French word meaning to *'to undertake or to do.'* Becoming a leader is within reach for anyone who wants to serve others and make a difference.

LEADERSHIP TODAY IS ABOUT INFLUENCE

> ***'The true measure of leadership is influence, nothing more nothing less'***
>
> ***– John C. Maxwell***

Leadership is defined as the capacity to influence people. *'Influence refers to one person's actual behaviour designed to change another person's attitudes, values, beliefs or behaviour.'* It is about making other people to get in accordance with your ideas, opinions and decisions. Influence allows leaders to get the things done; there can be no leadership without influence. Leadership is defined by a simple fact, *'how well you can influence your team across a series of roles and functions to meet organisational objectivs?'* The most important quality of a leader is to get along with others and influence their actions. For leaders, influence is like power and achieving more influence in the workplace is very important for success. Leadership is measured by influence; the greater your influences, the greater will be your leadership. Thus if you want to improve your leadership, you need to improve your influence. Today's leadership is more about influence and relationship than it is about control and giving orders.

Effective leaders help their team to understand how their contributions fit into the broader vision and inspire them to achieve the greater good of the organisation. Inspiration is not mandated, dictated or driven by authority. It is achieved by enlisting others, touching the hearts of team members while engaging their brains through the influence of leaders.

> ***The key to successful leadership today is influence, not authority.'***
>
> ***– Ken Blanchard***

LEADERSHIP AND MANAGEMENT

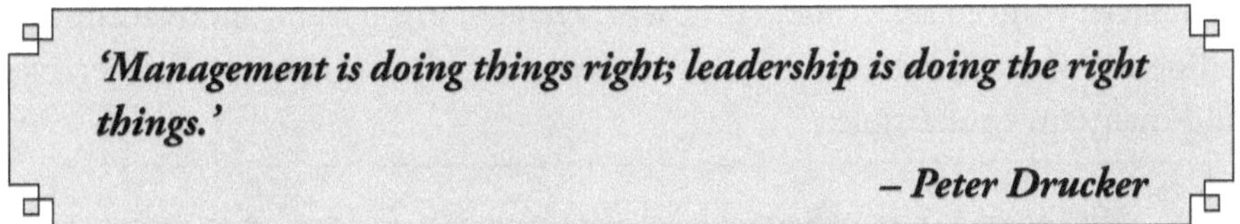

'Management is doing things right; leadership is doing the right things.'

– Peter Drucker

In an organisation, both managers and leaders take decisions, but there is a remarkable difference between them. Both roles are crucial, and they differ fundamentally. The words 'leader' and 'manager' are often used interchangeably; in fact, being a manager goes hand in hand with being a leader. The two must co-exist. Management skills are a subset of leadership skills; you cannot have one without the other. Leadership and management are two different and complementary concepts. Both are necessary for success. To become successful, you need to have capabilities in both areas. Both leadership and management are together required for task accomplishment.

The difference is in how the two approach the job via style and behaviour. For example, a manager tells the team members what to do, while a leader encourages them. A manager is a person in an organisation who is responsible for carrying out the four functions of management, including planning, organising, leading and controlling. Their primary concern is to accomplish organisational goals. Management is about getting things done through other people by creating an environment that enables them to give their best. A leader is *'a person who influences a group of people towards the achievement of a goal.'* Leadership refers to an individual's ability to influence, motivate, and enable others to contribute towards organisational success.

Leadership is different from management; perhaps the greatest separation between management and leadership is that leaders do not have to hold a management position. *'Everyone can lead,'* that is, a person can become a leader without a conventional title; i.e. leaders are leaders no matter what the title and the absence of title should not keep someone from leading. Leaders acquire their strength from within and not from a title or a position in the organisation. To build a truly outstanding organisation, every single person who works there must lead. Any individual can become a leader because the basis of leadership is on the personal qualities of the leader.

Management is a set of processes like planning, budgeting and staffing that keeps the organisation functioning; whereas leadership is about getting people to understand and believe in your vision and to work with you to achieve your goals. Leaders deal with change, inspiration, motivation and influence whereas managers deal with achieving the organisation's objectives and maintain equilibrium.

> ***'Management is efficiency in climbing the ladder of success. Leadership determines whether the ladder is leaning against the right wall.'***
>
> ***– Stephen R. Covey***

LEADERS AND MANAGERS

'Managers have the ability to get results; leaders have the vision for the future.'

– Brain Tracy

'Managers cope with change. Leaders cause it and make the competition change'

– John Kotler

'Managers help people to see themselves as they are. Leaders help people to see themselves better than they are.'

– Jim John

Leaders differ from managers in many dimensions and areas. Managers exercise control, while leaders create a system. Managers usually live by rules made by others; while leaders establish standards and then stick to them. Manager looks for the right fit between people and tasks whereas leaders look for the right fit between people and the vision. In practice, a leader can be a manager but a manager is not necessarily a leader. The basic difference between leaders and managers is that leaders have people follow them while managers have people who work for them. Here are some characteristics which separates leaders from managers.

Leaders don't have subordinates: Managers have subordinates and their power over others comes from formal authority. Leaders don't have subordinates, when they are leading. When they want to lead, they have to give up formal authoritarian control; because to lead is to have followers, and following is always a voluntary activity. *'Without followers a leader is not a leader.'*

> ***"Leadership is the art of getting someone else to do something you want done because he wants to do it."***
>
> ***– Dwight D. Eisenhower***

Leader creates leader: Managers don't have time to be bothered with concerns from their teams whereas leaders will look at their team members as humans, with potential to grow and get better. Understanding this, leaders will work to develop people into future leaders. For example; Swami Ramkrishna Paramahans through his kind touch had transferred all his spiritual powers to his successor Swami Vivekananda. Swami Vivekananda proved trustworthy and carried forward the message of his great master.

> ***'The function of leadership is to produce more leaders, not more followers.'***
>
> ***– Ralph Nader***

Leader is an innovator: A Leader is a person who is full of new ideas and believes in experimenting and creating new things. Every organisation needs transformational leaders, who believe in change, introduce change and push change. No stagnant organisation can survive in a competitive world. Leaders always work on taking the organisation ahead. Whereas, the manager is someone who is already established and is responsible for every organisational activity from top to bottom. He is the main control of the firm.

Leaders earn respect: According to Irwin Federman, *'your job gives you authority while your behaviour gets you respect.'* Respect is not something handed to you when you take on a new leadership role. It is an essential leadership quality that you must build over time. Leaders know that for team members to respect them, they need to earn it over time. Smart leaders work hard early on to earn the respect of their teams. Managers believe that title and authority will force others to respect them. When people respect you only because of your authority, they will give you the minimum effort.

> *'Respect is the key determinant of high performance. How much people respect you determine how well they perform.'*

Leaders give solutions: According to Brain Tracy, *'Leaders think and talk about the solutions. Followers think and talk about the problems.'* A leader will simply look at the problems and will devise new solutions to bring out the better by motivating team members whereas the manager will create policies for smooth functioning of the organisation. The mindset of the leader needs to be on the solution and not the problem.

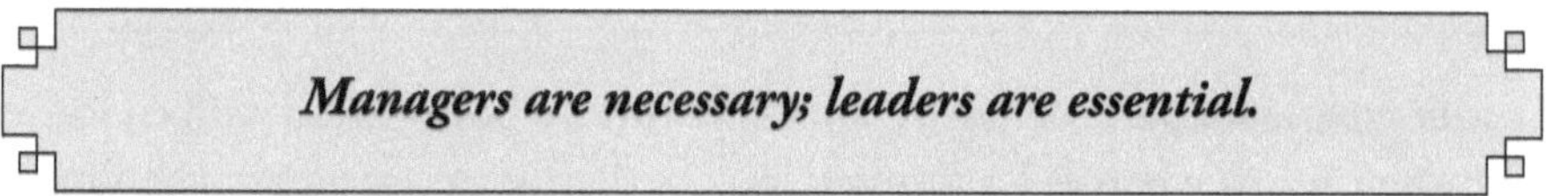

Managers are necessary; leaders are essential.

Manager vs Leader – Key Traits

Manager	Leader
A manager does things right	A leader does the right thing
Management is about efficiency	Leadership is about effectiveness
Implements directions from above; is generally in a reactive mode	Generates new ideas and directions; is generally in a proactive mode.
Directs people and enlists their cooperation	Motivates and inspires people to exceed their goals
Helps people cope with change	Helps people initiate change.
Improves skills of team members	Improves their attitudes and motivations
Managers have short term perspective	Leaders have long term perspective
Management is about how to do the things	Leadership is about what and why
Manager rely on control	Leader inspires trust
Manager relies on system	Leaders relies on people
Manager focuses on process and procedures	Leader focuses on vision and strategy

The position called 'manager' may not exist too much longer, and the concept of 'leadership' will be redefined. The twenty first century needs leaders not managers.

'Managers are for today. Leaders are for tomorrow. When you are a manager, people work for you. When you are a leader, you work for people.' Be a Leader not a boss or manager.

THE PHARMA FIRST-LINE LEADER

A pharma first-line leader is someone who is able to provide necessary skills to enable a group of medical representatives to achieve their objectives, to hold it together as a cohesive team and to motivate and develop them. The pharma first-line leader is the first link in the pharmaceutical sales management hierarchy. They are the extended arm of management and belong to the lower management; the employees (medical representatives) who report to them do not themselves have any managerial or supervisory responsibility. They are at the frontlines, and they make up 60% of a company's management ranks and directly supervise as much as 80% of the workforce i.e. medical representatives. First-line leaders are directly responsible for the day to day activities of medical representatives. They report to a second-line manager who is directly responsible for day to day activities of many teams each with one first-line leader. First-line leaders have to play an important role in driving the decision of senior management.

They handle medical representatives who generate revenue for the organisation. Their role is to plan, organise, execute and monitor the activities of medical representatives. They serve as role models for the medical representatives they supervise. They are the inspiration and guiding force to their medical representatives.

First-line leaders of tomorrow will have to establish a real vision and a sense of values for the organisation they wish to lead. They will have to communicate and motivate their medical representatives far more effectively than did the leaders in the past. ***Being a first-line leader is about serving your medical representatives and helping them succeed at their work.*** You have to remove all roadblocks in your medical representative's way.

People are constantly judging what other people do, say, or even what they wear, even if they don't verbalize their thoughts. The same is true in judging someone's ability to lead. No medical representatives want to follow their leaders blindly. They judge the strength of your leadership based on the signals they receive when interacting with you. If you present yourself in a professional manner, you will be perceived to have the qualities of an excellent first-line leader.

Skills of first-line leaders

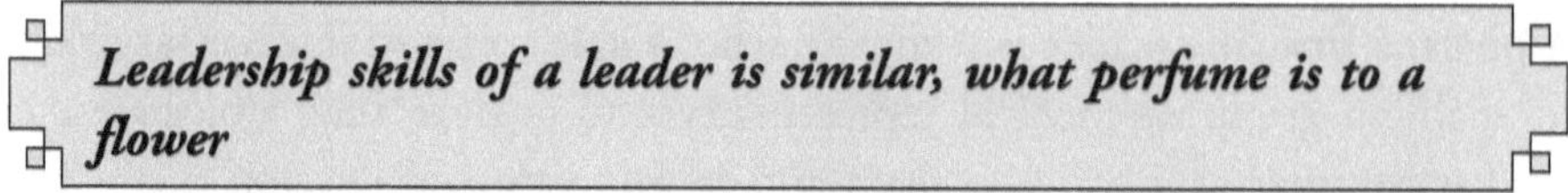

Leadership skills of a leader is similar, what perfume is to a flower

Every organisation needs leaders at every level. What makes people follow a leader? What makes a leader successful? The answer lies in the skills of a leader. All successful leaders possess some specific skills. These skills are the principle of leadership and play a huge role in your professional development. In fact, the leadership skills are same in any field of work. A pharmaceutical organisation is often only as good as its leader. If you want to elevate your company and your subordinates, you need to enhance your own character and skills first.

> ***'If you want to improve the organisation, you have to improve yourself and the organisation gets pulled up with you.'***
>
> ***– Indra Nooyi***

The skills of first-line leaders play an important role in development and performance of medical representatives. They require two sets of skills. The first set of skills is for delivering the business, which incorporates planning, organising, negotiation, decision-making, customer focus and commercial awareness. The second set of skills for dealing with medical representatives, which includes motivation, interpersonal skills, communication skills, and leadership. The more you display these skills, the more your medical representatives will believe and trust you. Below I have tried to explain some of the key skills that an effective first-line leader should possess.

1. Listening

Leadership begins with listening and *'The true leader is a listener.'* Leaders respect their team members by listening to them, as *'listening truly is the highest compliment.'* Listening is not just hearing as it involves both ear and brain. It is a skill that often has to be learned and practised. As a first-line leader, you must get passionate about understanding your team of medical representatives. Listening indicates that you trust the intelligence, skills and opinion of your team members. The most powerful way to connect with your medical representatives is to listen. Just listen. You first cultivate the skill of asking superb, open ended questions and then listen to them. The questions are designed to get your medical representatives to open up and connect with you. Asking questions goes hand in hand with listening.

> ***'One of the most sincere forms of respect is actually listening to what another has to say.'***
>
> ***– Bryant H. McGill***

2. Communication

The word which is most closely associated with leadership is communication. A leader can accomplish nothing unless he or she can communicate effectively. A good leader is a good communicator. Communication is not *'what you say.'* It is also *'how you say.'* Communication is not just the actual word you use; it is much more. All round communication involves verbal words, eye contacts, facial expressions, posters, gestures etc. The greater part of your message made up of non-verbal hints/signals, tone of voice and listening. Developing excellent communication skills is absolutely essential to effective leadership. As a leader, you must get things done through medical representatives therefore you must have the ability to inspire and motivate, guide, direct and listen. It's only through effective communication that you can create substantial positive change and influence your medical representatives to internalise their vision and implement it.

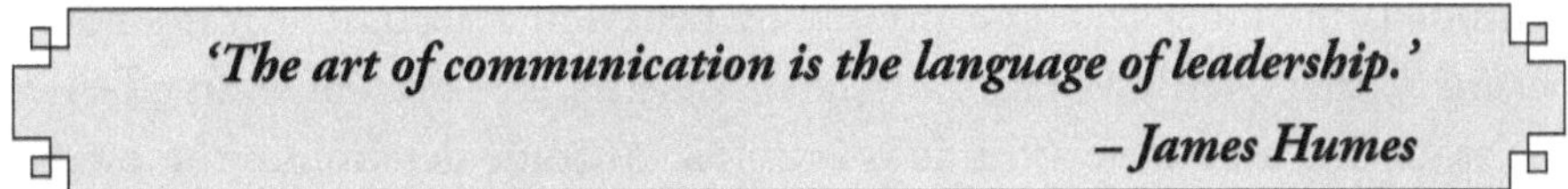

> ***'The art of communication is the language of leadership.'***
>
> ***– James Humes***

3. Passion

Passion is an intense emotion, a compelling enthusiasm or desire for something. What makes it possible for people who might seem ordinary to achieve great things? The answer is passion. Nothing can take the place of passion in leader's life. Passion is contagious. Watching a passionate leader energises the entire organisation. Passion generates a supply of positive energy for the first-line leaders. It is the passion, which increases their ability to impact on medical representatives. *'A leader with great passion and few skills always outperforms a leader with great skills and no passion.'*

> ***'A great leader's courage to fulfil his vision comes from passion, not position.'***
>
> ***– John C. Maxwell***

4. Empathy

Empathy is the experience of understanding another person's condition from their perspective. Empathy means *'putting yourself in the other person's shoes'* and is evident in the statement *'Your pain in my heart.'* The ability to have and display empathy is an important part of leadership. Studies reveal that the empathy is positively related to job performance. It is essential for you to understand the medical representative's world fully and to let them know that you understand it. If you are an empathetic leader, you will care for your medical representatives and as a result they will feel valued and appreciated. Empathy fosters positive feelings, and is fundamental to effective leadership.

> ***'When dealing with people, remember you are not dealing with creatures of logic, but with creatures of emotion.'***
>
> ***– Dale Carnegie***

5. Positive Attitude

Attitude is the inner feeling expressed by behaviour. Attitude is really how a person is, that overflows into how he or she acts. For becoming an effective leader, having a positive attitude is essential. Attitude determines the success and failure for a leader. The difference between an obstacle and an opportunity is simply the attitude of a leader towards it. According to William James, *'the greatest discovery of my generation is that people can alter their lives by altering their attitudes of minds.'* Effective pharma first-line leaders must have a positive attitude that is upbeat and courageous. Positive attitude can lift the spirits of the team and can inspire them to keep pressing on until they succeed. It is the endeavour of a positive first-line leader to transform negative thoughts into positive orientations. If you have a positive attitude, then nothing can stop you from achieving your goals.

> ***'Leadership is practised not so much in words as in attitude and in actions.'***
>
> ***– Harold S. Geneen***

6. Integrity

Integrity is the most valuable and respected quality of leadership. It is the quality of being honest and having strong moral principles which makes people trust you. Integrity in a leader is a concept of consistency of actions, values, methods, measures, principles, expectations and outcomes. Integrity is defined as the consistency between what a leader says and what the leader does. In fact, *'integrity is doing the right thing when no one is watching.'* A leader has no chance of being perceived as a great leader in the long run if his or her integrity comes into question. Great leaders have integrity. Pharma first-line leaders with integrity are trusted by their medical representatives. Mutual trust between you and medical representatives is very important, once it is lost; it is very difficult to re-establish it.

> ***'It is true that integrity alone won't make you a leader, but without integrity you will never be one.'***
>
> ***– Zig Zaglar***

7. Vision

Vision is a clear, distinctive and specific view of the future. *'Vision is the art of seeing what is invisible to others.'* We all have a vision for something, but great leaders not only have vision but also have the trait of transferring their vision to the team members so that it becomes an organisational vision. Vision is indispensable because vision leads the leader and draws him forward. Success of a leader always starts with vision. Vision is a powerful tool for a first-line leader that drives the performances of medical representatives. With a vision and a plan success is only a step away. Vision sets the direction and purpose. Vision inspires enthusiasm, belief and commitment of the medical representatives. In order to make your vision into reality you will need belief in your idea, and you should consider how to protect as well as play to the strengths of your medical representatives. There is saying, *'only when you dream it, you can do it.'*

To be successful; dream big, have a vision in mind and sincerely work towards realising that vision.

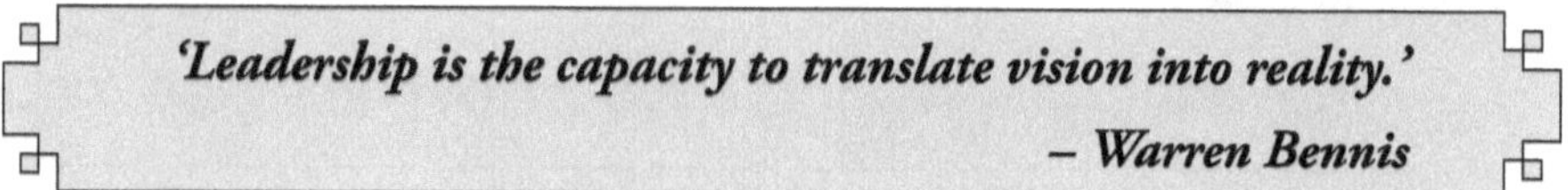

'Leadership is the capacity to translate vision into reality.'

– Warren Bennis

8. Initiative

Initiative is defined as work behaviour characterised by its self-starting in nature. Initiative is doing the right thing without being told and it's a proactive approach. Taking the initiative is a crucial element of leadership. Initiative makes a person stand apart from the crowd and transforms into a leader. The best leaders are proactive. They don't wait for someone else to tell them what to do. If you want to become an effective leader, you must be willing to initiate and put yourself on the line. An effective leader with initiative looks for opportunities and makes the best use of them. If you can think, introspect and practice the habit of forethought, you can develop initiative. Taking initiative by a first-line leader is an infectious enthusiasm for medical representatives.

'Without initiative, leaders are simply workers in leadership positions.'

9. Innovation

Today's world is constantly being innovated with new ideas and technology and all these are based on finding new solutions for the same problems. Innovative means trying new things; and in current scenario, all leaders constantly flex their minds and elevate their abilities by consistently asking themselves *'what I can improve today?'* They have a deeply held commitment to make everything they touch better than they found it, and to constantly reinvent themselves along the way. That's the essence of innovation. *'Leadership needs to not only think different, but they need to act different.'* What separates creative leaders from non-creative leaders is their ability to generate and execute innovative ideas. Without innovation, pharmaceutical organisations are likely to struggle.

'Innovation distinguishes between a leader and a follower.'

– Steve Jobs

10. Mental Toughness

This is an important skill a leader requires in dealing with challenges and changes in the working environment. Leaders who display characteristics of mental toughness flourish within the world of work. They set high standards, and they will not accept anything but the best. Mental toughness implies deep commitment to a moral principle and also an indication of more being demanding in terms of the common task. Mental toughness should always be expressed in the context of fairness. First-line leaders need to be tough or demanding but fair. They need to be even-handed in their demands on medical representatives.

> ***'Toughness is in the soul and spirit, not in muscles.'***
>
> ***– Alex Karras***

11. Courage

'Courage is the mark of greatness in leadership'

According to Jim Mellado, *'Leadership is the expression of courage that compels people to do the right thing.'* Whenever we see significant progress in an organisation, it is quite obvious that the leaders made courageous decisions. Willingness to take risk is common in highly effective leaders. There is a saying that FEAR is an acronym for *'False Expectations Appearing Real.'* Fear is the biggest enemy in one's success. Courage is not absence of fear, it's doing what you are afraid to do. You should do the thing you fear, your fear will disappear. In pharmaceutical business, courageous action is really a special kind of calculated risk-taking. Courage is the ability of a first-line leader to do what needs to be done, regardless of the cost or risk. It is the courage of the first-line leaders that causes medical representatives to associate around the banner of them.

> ***'Courage is the first virtue that makes all other virtues possible.'***
>
> ***– Aristotle***

12. Humility

Humility is the most important quality of a leader. Humility can be simply defined as not believing that you are superior to others and this helps leaders to get rid of their egos while leading. Humility is not a weakness, rather it is strength. Humility is actually the trait that magnifies all other positive traits. Without humility all of a leader's other strengths become diminished. Great leaders are humble and a sense of humility is very essential to leadership. Humility makes first-line leaders approachable; which enables them to connect with their medical representatives. First-line leaders who practice humility engender trust and empower their medical representatives. Humble leaders are more effective and better liked.

> ***'Great leaders don't need to act tough; their humility serves to underscores their toughness.'***
>
> ***– Simon Sinek.***

13. Enthusiasm

Enthusiasm is considered as the secret of success. When it comes to leadership, enthusiasm can often be more important than other skills. Enthusiasm is as important as hard work. Enthusiasm is a strong feeling of active interest in something which actually drives passion and fuels achievement. It comes from within. Enthusiasm is demonstrated by having a sense of urgency. Enthusiasm is infectious and makes leaders more credible. Twenty first century needs enthusiastic leadership. Enthusiastic first-line leaders are able to make visions come alive, and it becomes contagious among medical representatives. It's the enthusiastic transmission of energy that brings a vision to life for the medical representatives.

> ***'Enthusiasm is the mother of effort, and without it nothing great was ever achieved.'***
>
> ***– Ralph Waldo Emerson***

KEY POINTS: Leadership Skills

1. *Knowledge of leadership skills will not make you a leader.*
2. *Leadership demands no special education; it requires a lot of practice and a genuine willingness to learn.*
3. *Leadership skills are interconnected. If you start practicing one skill, others will slowly develop their own.*
4. *You can start practicing with any skill because these skills belong to a circle, where every point is a starting point as well as an ending point.*
5. *Leaders never stop developing their skills. They are lifelong students. Always aim to develop your leadership skills to create optimum results.*

"Leadership is experiential; it's really a trained art." Leadership requires lots of study and practice to become skilled.

Nobody is a born leader. One needs to develop leadership skills. If you want to become a leader, remember that it's in your mind. ***'To become a leader, you need to think like a leader; to think like a leader you have to act like a leader.'*** Once you understand how to think like a leader, it will become easier to act like a leader. Also it is very essential to dress in a professional manner when you do so.

Many of the world's most strong leaders have several skills in common. Understanding the skills of strong leaders and cultivating those skills is useful for those pursuing a career in pharmaceutical selling.

Adversity Builds Great Leaders

Most people hide in their shells when the going gets tough. They push away anything that pulls them the least bit out of their comfort zone. By doing so, they also push away their chances for growth, mastery and lasting achievement. 'When you go to your limits, your limits will expand'; this means the more time you spend in the discomfort zone, the more your comfort zone will expand. Difficult days never last, but tough people always do.

Adversity or crisis is inevitable. As a leader, the only thing that matters is how you deal with it when it comes.

The true test of leadership is how well you function in adverse situations; adversity reveals a leader's character. Adversity makes a first-line leader wise.

The adversities are nothing more than chances to become heroic, similarly the true character of a leader shines through in adversity. A leader's competencies are tested during a crisis. Leaders often emerge from crises. Several great leaders in world history attained height during adverse situations. Great leaders relish a challenge. They wait for the opportunity to test their skills and prove their real mettle. The adverse conditions can actually elevate the skills of a leader and also a leader can show his hidden talent.

Let us consider the example of Saurav Ganguly, one of the most successful captains of the Indian cricket team. Ganguly has demonstrated very effectively all the qualities of a corporate leader. He took charge of the team at a time when Indian cricket was in crisis because of the match fixing controversy. He demonstrated that great leaders turn crisis into opportunity. He believed, imparted self-belief in his team members and set about raising the bar. Leadership is all about the capacity to manage with complexity. He brought in all the skills required to hold over the crisis and rebuilt the Indian team into a unit which could conquer the world.

'The quality of a leader is reflected in the standards they set for themselves.'

In Pharmaceutical business, when the competition is weak and the customers are loyal then anyone can be a star. Difficult times are one that reveals what you're made of and what kind of leader you actually are. Difficult times are the best opportunities to show leadership. Followings are some of the tips in dealing with crisis:

1. *Stay cool, don't get angry.*
2. *Believe in yourself, you can handle it.*
3. *Before taking any decision, find out exactly what has happened.*
4. *Take charge, make a plan and keep your team members informed.*
5. *Never give up, persist until you succeed.*

'A smooth sea never made a skilled sailor.'

Role, Responsibilities and Accountabilities

When we think about the roles, the first thing that strikes our mind is the role of an actor or actress in a film. Like in films, roles are played in real life also. In an organisation, everyone has a role to play. A 'ROLE' is a set behaviour associated with a particular position or designation in an organisation. In order to perform the roles, a leader needs certain skills, that is, the ability to perform the roles effectively. The success depends on how well you know your roles and how effectively you play them.

Responsibility comes from the Latin word 'responsus' which means 'to respond.' Responsibility is the ability and authority to act or decide on one's own without supervision; it gives people a feeling of belonging and ownership. In other words, responsibility is your ability to respond to a situation. Responsibility of a person means the work or duties assigned to him by virtue of his position in the organisation. Leadership is taking responsibility.

'Responsibility is the obligation to carry out assigned activities to the best of his abilities.'

– George Terry

Accountability is defined as willingness to accept responsibility which means is a state of being accountable, liable or answerable. Being accountable simply means being responsible for decisions made, actions taken, and completion of the assignments. Accountability is crucial in ensuring high performance within an organisation. However, leaders must clearly communicate their expectations to the person who is responsible for the specified action or task. Clear communication of expectations and well defined goals is a very effective tool in enhancing performance at every level of organisation.

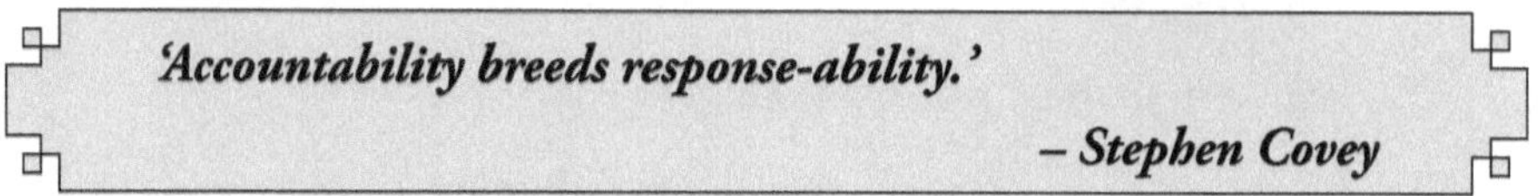

> ***'Accountability breeds response-ability.'***
>
> ***– Stephen Covey***

The main difference between responsibility and accountability is that responsibility can be shared while accountability cannot. If you are accountable for something, you are in a position that requires you to report to or answer to someone for your actions and decisions. If you are responsible for something, you may be the one to whom things are reported.

To lead a team of medical representatives, first-line leaders should have enough clarity not only about their roles and responsibilities but also about the medical representatives. Let us familiarise with the roles, responsibilities and accountabilities of a medical representative which will enable us to understand those of a first-line leader.

Role of Medical Representatives

- To meet all doctors in his assigned territory, as per frequency stipulated by the company.
- To follow the strategy/discipline laid down by the company.
- To prepare and regularly update the list of doctors, retailers from the territory assigned.
- They need to provide the market feedback to the company.
- They should provide professional services to the doctor as per the system of the company.
- They keep the company informed by sending activity and results reports, such as daily call reports, weekly work plans, and monthly and annual territory analysis.

Responsibilities of Medical Representatives

- The prime responsibilities of medical representatives are 'Prescription Generation.'
- Doctor list preparation is the shared responsibilities of a Medical representative and first-line leader, but the accountability of the correctness of the list is that of the first-line leader.
- Selection of the right product for the right doctors (Brand Matrix) is the prime responsibility.
- Carrying out RCPA (retail chemist prescription audit) is a very important responsibility.
- Checking inventory at the stockiest level, placing orders and realising payments.
- Building the company's image in their respective territories.

Accountability of medical representatives

Through prescription generation, the Medical Representative has to complete the sales objectives set by the company, product wise as well as value wise every month and also month after month.

Transition to Management from Medical Representative

First-line managers are the strongest model for the medical representatives. Often the first-line managers are promoted from the ranks of medical representatives based on their performance as individual contributors. However, the best individual contributor doesn't always make the best manager. The fact is management skills are very different from the skills one needs to succeed as an individual contributor. Once you are promoted as a first-line manager, it is important to remember that your job is not to sell; it is to help medical representatives sell more and sell more easily.

The transition from individual contributor to management represents a profound psychological adjustment; as transformation as managers contend with new responsibilities. There is a transition in the mindset as well as in the roles. They are pushed from a place of I, me and mine to we, us and ours. Getting this transition right accelerates your career trajectory.

'When you become a leader, you lose the right to think about yourself.'

– Gerald Brooks

As you undergo the transition to manager, you need to separate your personal relationship from professional one. You also need your interpersonal behavioural modification to adapt to different people or subordinates not expecting them to adapt every time. ***This is the secret of Leadership.*** *When you become a manager, you become a part of management. Your previous personal relationships with co-workers will need to be moved to a different level because you're no longer a medical representative; you are now the person who assigns work, analyses productivity and provides performance appraisals.*

To be a manager, you'll need to shift your focus and acquire a whole new set of skills. Newly promoted managers must learn how to lead others, to win trust and respect, to motivate and to strike the right balance between delegation and control. They must learn the differences between managing individual performance and the performance of their teams. Remember, your position as the new manager isn't about trying to be popular; it's about leading others to achieve results. And most first-line managers find it difficult to make the transition; some never do.

The skills needed to succeed as a medical representative and those needed to be effective as a first-line manager are completely different. Once you become first- line manager; you have to get the job done by medical representatives. Most importantly your performance will be judged on the performance of your medical representatives. To become a successful first-line leader, it is imperative to align the aspiration of medical representatives with the goals of the organisation.

KEY POINTS: How to Make a Smoother Transition to Management?

1. *When you become a manager, accept the job change; change your attitude.*
2. *Focus on your medical representatives; they don't work for you. You work for them.*
3. *Ensure each medical representative has everything they need to succeed.*
4. *Invest time in making each medical representative as capable as you were.*
5. *Ask for honest feedback, this will help you learn and refine your leadership style.*

'Before you become a leader, success is about growing yourself, and when you become a leader, success is about growing others.'

–Jack Welch

Being a leader is a never ending journey as there are many roles that a leader has to acquire. Followings are the roles, responsibilities and accountabilities of a first-line leader:

Role of first-line leaders

- The main role is to build up a team of medical representatives.
- Utilisation of organisational resources to accomplish objectives.

- Elaborate organisation's vision and mission to the internal and external clients.
- To ensure that the prescription share of your brands are increased by getting the strategies implemented by the medical representative.
- To create 'core customers' and to retain them to continue the business and growth in the assigned area.
- First-line leaders should have direct contact with the key doctors and retailers in their area. They need to build trust and confidence among the key doctors as well as ensure the business.

Responsibilities of first-line leaders

- First-line leaders are responsible for organising, planning, directing and controlling the activities of medical representatives.
- Strategy execution and to ensure that medical representatives stay one stage ahead.
- They have to create a vision that is compelling enough to motivate medical representatives towards attaining organisational goals.
- They have to develop and coach his medical representatives.
- Generate enthusiasm and keep the team motivated and energised.
- They have to build relations with KOL and leading retailers.
- Appraise their medical representatives.

Shared responsibilities of medical representative and first-line leader

- Along with medical representatives first-line leaders have shared responsibilities of the preparation of the doctor list.
- Ensure the correctness of doctor-product match through retail prescription audits.
- Availability of all products at all the retailers.

Accountabilities of first-line leaders

- Accountable for successful implementation of company's strategies.
- Ensuring correctness of doctors list being met by medical representatives.
- Accountable for achieving budgets, medical representative-wise, product wise etc.
- First-line leaders are accountable for success of new product launches.

> ***'First-line leaders should possess right attitude, good communication skills with leadership qualities, and should be capable of building an energetic team with a competitive edge and ability to execute the plan for achievement of pre-decided organisational goals'***

Three Primary Activities

The success of first-line leaders is measured by their effectiveness in leading the team of medical representatives. They need to be good communicators, with the ability to build rapport, set goals, make decisions and solve problems. The first-line leadership process is consists of three primary activities:

1. Pharmaceutical Sales Management
2. Strategy Execution
3. Development of Medical Representative

The quality of execution of all these activities depends on the skill-levels that first-line leaders have developed in each area.

1. Pharmaceutical Sales Management

Medical representatives of the pharmaceutical organisation meet the doctor and promote their product through visual aid, clinical paper presentation or sample distribution. Medical representatives try to influence prescription patterns of doctors in favour of their brands. Based on the presentation made and the confidence gained by the doctor, the product is prescribed by the doctor to a patient.

The patient purchases the product from the chemist. This is termed as a sale in Pharmaceutical selling.

Pharmaceutical marketing is a specialised field where medical representatives form the backbone of the entire marketing effort. Pharmaceutical marketing is a process which identifies, anticipates and satisfies doctor's needs at a profit.

Sales management is the functional process for planned and efficient utilisation of resources to get the desired results. It is the process of generating sales that are essential to the survival of the organization. The role of sales managers is to achieve sales by working with and through their team members. Pharmaceutical sales management is a cluster of activities which includes doctor list preparation, specific brand promotion, territory management, doctor conversion, directing and controlling medical representatives etc. Pharmaceutical sales management is tough one as it is associated with hurdles, challenges and disappointments. The results are often not commensurate with efforts. Sales management, like any other job, can be learned.

Selling is a lot more than telling. The new approach to selling is about building relationships and trust. The pharmaceutical sales management is an on-going process which involves relationship-building through trust and doctor satisfaction developed over a long period of time.

First-line leaders are the key to pharmaceutical sales management because they have more influence on the level of sales and ultimately, the level of profitability of the organization. They supervise all the activities associated with sales management. They spend 90% of their time with the medical representatives. They must be able to spot opportunities, create new approaches to interact with doctors in a way that differentiates them from competition and connects them to doctors meaningfully.

Following are the elements of sales management:

Doctor list preparation – Each medical representative has a list of potential doctors, and the first-line leaders are accountable for the correctness of the list. To prepare a correct list of doctors, you need to guide your medical representatives in collecting following information:

- Name, address and qualification.

- Specialty of the doctor – Find out if he is GP, CP, surgeon, etc. *'The thumb rule is to go by practice not by qualification.'*
- Size of Practice – Find out the number of patients per day.
- Category – Whether attached to Govt., Semi Govt. or private hospitals.
- Type of Patients – The patients may belong to middle, poor or upper class. This determines the buying capacities of patients.

The most important source of collecting the above information is the chemist. The retail chemist can provide information of trade doctors; however, for hospital and nursing home doctors, the source of information is the pharmacist or the purchasing authority attached to the hospital. The case records in the indoor wards also provide a lot of information.

Correct brand matrix: This is nothing but different products for different doctors to get better results. Medical representatives prepare a list of doctors and divides their products among the doctors. The brand matrix makes the call effective and productive. The brand matrix allows doctors to listen, takes interest, clarifies doubts if any and helps the doctor feel relaxed enough to make a commitment. You must guide your medical representatives how to target right product to the right doctors. You need to demonstrate how to do an 'Rx audit' or 'brand review' at the chemist level so that medical representative asks the right question to the chemist. For example:

- For a particular composition, which are largest selling brands?
- Who are the doctors prescribing those brands?
- How many prescriptions given by each doctor per week or month?

Based on the above information, medical representatives find out the potentiality of a doctor for a particular brand and decide the brand for that doctor accordingly. Your success depends on how accurately you assess the potentiality in preparing a correct brand matrix.

Territory management: A medical representative is given some geographical area to cover, to do all the activities to sell and to promote sales. This is called Territory. Territory management is a process that allows medical representatives to achieve their objectives from the potential doctors in a given geographic area. Normally a territory consists of 'Headquarter' (The place where the medical representative is based) and the 'Ex or out station' (the places to be covered from the headquarter). Headquarter is a place where maximum numbers of customers are located. You have to ensure that your medical representatives have a thorough knowledge of their territories. For example, the medical representative must know the followings:

- Map and geography of the territory.
- Major towns with their status, i.e. District, Sub division or any special place.
- Mode of transport, distances and time taken to reach different locations from his base town.
- Key players in the territory in terms of distributors, important retailers, etc.
- Market information including doctors, their status, and prescription habits, etc.

For successful territory management, you have to ensure that your medical representative covers all the listed doctors as per the frequency pattern designed by the company. You need to prepare STP and Fare charts for your team members.

STP, i.e. standard tour programme is a fixed tour plan for the entire financial year to ensure regular coverage of all the listed doctors with predetermined frequency. The STP should be prepared for 24 working days. Based on the STP, the medical representative prepares a monthly tour plan which you have to approve. While preparing the fare chart, the objective should be to achieve customer coverage in the most economical manner possible.

First-line leaders play the role of a business manager while preparing the fare chart for medical representatives. Based on the potential, they identify the towns to be covered once in a month and towns to be covered twice or thrice in a month. With the distances and mode of transport, they prepare and review the fare chart for medical representatives. Fare chart helps better planning and rationalising the expense.

Doctor conversion: The health of a pharmaceutical organisation is related to the prescriptions that medical representatives able to generate. Conversion of a doctor is a challenging task that calls for sincere efforts, regular visits to doctors and chemists/stockists, proper use of promotional inputs including literature and samples of medicines and strict adherence to the work norms laid down by the Company. Always let doctors to make the decision to prescribe. You have to ensure that your medical representatives do this by asking questions to the doctors and steering the conversation until doctors realise that your product is the solution they have been looking for.

Conversation with doctors is the bridge between doctor and Rx

However, conversion of a doctor is a single act, but a long term procedure. You rarely achieve instant success with one call. The reason is as follows –

- Prescription potential can only be developed gradually.
- Prescription habit of the doctor is hard to break. The change from the use of one drug to another takes time.
- Each call brings the medical representative closer to his/her long term objective. In practice, each call achieves part of the objective.

In pharmaceutical sales, the effectiveness of a call depends on competences of a medical representative. Medical representatives must be well equipped with product knowledge which involves intensive study of pharmacology, anatomy and physiology in order to convert a doctor or to generate prescriptions. You need to train and equip them so that they can convert doctors and can generate prescriptions. Also, you need to ensure that the medical representative must convert new doctors for his existing brands to counter competitors effectively. If they don't create new prescribers in a competitive market, you will face deterioration in sales when competitors convert your prescribers.

Conversion of doctor requires a great deal of salesmanship. Salesmanship is defined as *'The science of understanding human desires and pointing the way to their fulfilment.'* Anybody in this world who sells products, services or ideas is a salesman. Selling is an art because it involves human interaction; selling is science as it follows a certain series of steps. Salesmanship is a combination of both art and science. Successful salesmanship is 90% preparation and 10% presentation. You have to develop the salesmanship of your medical representatives so that they convert new doctors and maintain a pipeline of future doctors. Conversion of doctors is an on-going process.

Engage your medical representatives in more activities – *'The law of probability says that if you engage in more activities aimed at generating sales, you will ultimately generate more sales.'* One of the quickest ways to increase sales is to increase sales activities. In our context, for example, there is a direct relationship between the number of doctors a medical representative visits and the sales he or she generates. You have to motivate your team members to do more doctor calls. You have to monitor the call average and keep them informed regularly.

Provide clear direction to medical representatives – According to John Maxwell, *'a leader is one who knows the way, goes the way and shows the way.'* The medical representatives generate revenue as well as carry the future profits of the organisation on their backs. Where do they turn to for direction, motivation, and support? The answer, of course, is the first-line leader who is charged with providing the insights, supports, and motivating medical representatives so that they can succeed. Medical representatives need and frequently look for direction when they do not have knowledge, skills or capabilities to accomplish a task or to achieve an objective. Without providing a clear vision and steps to get there, you won't be able to keep your medical representatives motivated.

In practice, first-line leaders should be like veteran tour guides who take people along with them to places, they know thoroughly. They need to be present throughout the process both physically and mentally, guiding, teaching and sharing their passion about each place that they visit.

> ***Delegation and direction are both part of the management equation. However, too much direction, on the other hand, can demotivate a medical representative.***

2. Strategy Execution

> ***First-line leaders are the bridge between strategy and execution.***

A strategy is a business approach, a set of competitive moves that are designed to generate a successful outcome through systematic working at doctor and chemist levels. A strategy is a comprehensive master planning, through which a pharmaceutical organisation can achieve success in the market. ***Strategy gives direction to the organisation.***

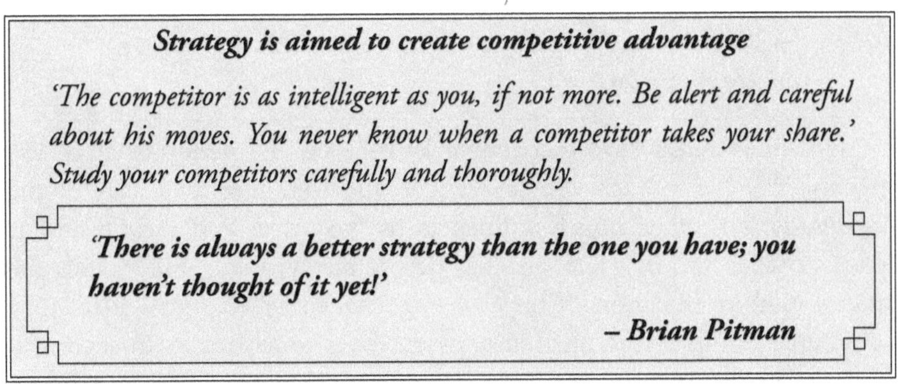

Strategy is aimed to create competitive advantage

'The competitor is as intelligent as you, if not more. Be alert and careful about his moves. You never know when a competitor takes your share.' Study your competitors carefully and thoroughly.

> ***'There is always a better strategy than the one you have; you haven't thought of it yet!'***
>
> ***– Brian Pitman***

For a strategy to be successful it must be executed. The draft of a strategy is like the architect's plan for new buildings, not real until it is built. Execution of a strategy means, transforming the strategies into actions to achieve the objectives. However, translating strategy into action is tougher than it sounds. It has been found that 90% of organisations fail to execute on their strategies. Strategy execution has become a challenge around the world due to its staggering high failure rate.

> ***'Good strategies never fail; they fail because we do not know how to execute them.'***

First-line leader is the custodian of the strategies; in fact, the bridge between strategy and its execution is the first-line leader. They have a fundamental responsibility to create the right condition for execution. They must stay focused on the execution and make sure that medical representatives are taking the right actions. It is the first-line leadership who must motivate and direct medical representatives to execute the strategies.

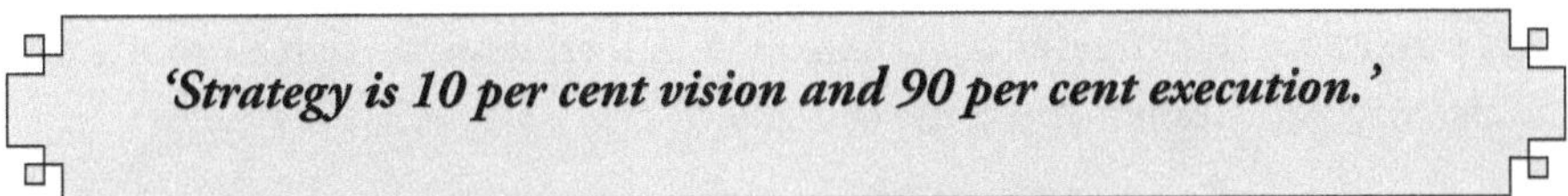

> ***'Strategy is 10 per cent vision and 90 per cent execution.'***

For example; if the strategy is that the medical representatives must meet VVIP doctors three times in a month, the first-line leader must guide them so that they meet those VVIP doctors as per the frequency. The level of execution must make the distinction between effective and non-effective leaders.

> ***'Without strategy, execution is aimless; without execution, strategy is useless'***

First-line leaders have exceptional leverage on the performance of the organisation. How much conviction and understanding they have of the organisation's strategy, hugely influences the way they lead their teams. It is very crucial that first-line leader is deeply involved and understands the strategy and its execution. If they are engaged, energised, and skilled, they communicate this to the medical representatives which results in successful execution of the strategy.

However, strategy often fails because the first-line leaders do not focus on aligning their medical representatives to the strategies of their organisation. Strategy execution is not done by telling the medical representative what to do, rather sharing the strategy in a way that everyone can understand and buy into it, and see how their jobs relate to it. For a successful execution; the key requirements of a first-line leader are:

Make medical representative understands the strategy: One of the most pressing challenges in all of strategy is simply understanding the strategy. You have to ensure that each of your medical representatives understand it properly. You must communicate the strategy to them in a way that will help them understand not only what needs to be done, but why. In fact, you have to sell strategy to your medical representatives.

Enable and motivate medical representatives: You need to keep on motivating your medical representatives to execute the strategies. You must create a culture of trust and commitment that motivates medical representatives to execute the strategy. Continually tell your medical representatives how good they are and what a great job they are doing. When a medical representative feels motivated the strategy gets implemented more easily.

Serve as an example: Set an example in everything you do; because your medical representatives are watching what you are doing and what you are saying. Your behaviour will guide the behaviour of your team members. You must set an example of the behaviours, skills and attitudes that are required by the strategy.

Follow up: A follow up is a further observation or monitoring of the on-going assignments in order to increase its effectiveness. Leadership is also about following up on those tasks and making sure they are done to your team members. You need to keep a regular follow up on the progress of the strategy; give regular feedback and offer additional support when required. Periodic follow up helps to keep medical representatives on the track.

Give recognition: In strategy execution also, what gets measured gets done and what gets measured and rewarded gets done faster. Every medical representative looks for recognition if not reward; you need to appreciate immediately. Recognition should be given formally or informally. To be of any value, recognition has to be genuine and sincere. Giving recognition publicly reinforces it.

3. Development of Medical Representative

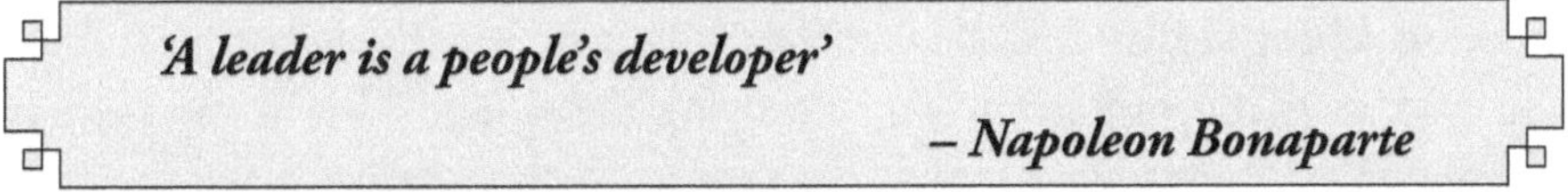

'A leader is a people's developer'

– Napoleon Bonaparte

Medical representatives are the most valuable asset for the first-line leaders. Development of a medical representative is the most important and rewarding thing a first-line leader can do. It is your moral responsibility to develop medical representatives because their efforts and output ultimately determine the performance and will further push you up.

> *'A leader becomes great, not because of their power, but because of their ability to empower others.'*

Find what is good about medical representatives and do everything you can to illuminate their work, support their development and nurture their success. When you develop medical representatives, they become smarter, more productive and they perform on a higher level. You Should:

Set an example – Leaders are leaders because of their actions and through their actions they set examples in the workplace. Examples are very important because medical representatives take in information more through their eyes than their ears. Remember you are a source of inspiration of your team. Medical representatives take their cues from their first-line leaders; therefore, it is important for you to behave the way you expect them to behave. You must have to ensure that your words and actions must go together – they should support each other. Medical representatives are looking to you, watching for clues and modelling your style. For example, if you want your medical representatives to be better disciplined, more organized and punctual, you must raise the bar on yourself. You must become better disciplined, more organized and more punctual.

Develop sense of belonging – *'When an employee has a sense of belonging in the workplace, it connotes ownership.'* Medical representatives who feel like they belong will stay in their jobs longer, collaborate better and can go the extra mile. You have to ensure that each medical representative should develop a sense of belongingness with the organisation. This will also create a feeling of ownership among them. There are different ways by which you can foster the sense of belongingness of your medical representatives. For example; a sense of belonging comes from a genuine effort in investing time in your medical representatives, involving them in decision-making etc.

Develop selling skills – Excellent selling skills is an essential factor for success. You have to spend more time on improving the selling skills of the medical representative. Never assume that the medical representatives have mastered the essential selling skills. First, you must identify the skill that needs to develop in your medical representative. The next step is to teach the skill, its purpose, and how to perform it properly. This may require multiple training sessions to complete. Once the medical representative is able to perform the skill properly, you must motivate and coach them to use it repeatedly. Development is not complete until appropriate utilisation of the skill in an internalised habit that is performed unconsciously.

'Selling skills are not tricks and tactics, but techniques and principles.'

Provide opportunities for professional and personal growth – Organisations grow when the people inside them grow first. Growth is a huge motivational factor in engagement of medical representatives. To ensure continuous growth and improve productivity; equip them with the tools they need to function at peak performance. You have to ensure that the medical representatives take on new challenges, expand their capabilities, cultivate new behaviours and entertain new ideas.

Become a mentor – Mentoring facilitates your medical representatives to excel beyond expectation. As a mentor you must share your own personal experiences, insights and knowledge with the medical representatives. Today's medical representatives are the future leaders. It is your duty to make them leaders. Help your medical representatives to gain leadership skills. Develop them so that they can lead themselves. Medical representatives should feel that they are leaders and are supposed to act as leaders.

When you help your medical representatives to think about how they could do better in future, they feel happy about you and about their job. Empower your medical representatives to perform at their best by continually reminding them how good they are and how much you believe in them.

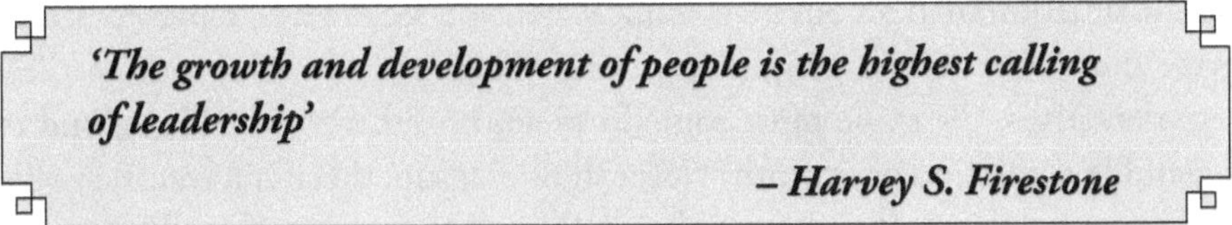

'The growth and development of people is the highest calling of leadership'
– Harvey S. Firestone

How to deal with Medical Representatives

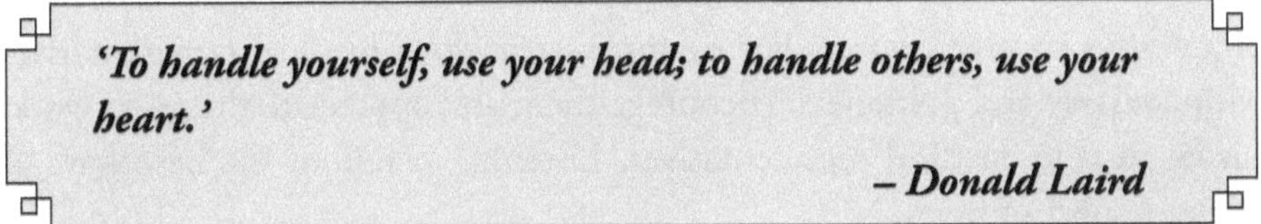

'To handle yourself, use your head; to handle others, use your heart.'
– Donald Laird

The success of any person in any field depends on other people. Regardless of the physical or financial assets we may or may not have, it's people who make us successful. Dealing with people successfully is an art and is the essential ingredient for success in business. Studies have shown that 85% of success is due to the ability to deal with people successfully. Leadership is about people; all leaders need to deal with people. The success of a first-line leader depends on medical representatives. You cannot achieve any success without taking your medical representatives into account. If you want to be successful, you need to learn to deal with your medical representatives. Following are some of the tips of dealing with medical representatives:

Make a good impression – Making a good impression is essential to becoming an influential leader. The best way is to let your medical representatives know that you are impressed by them. Every encounter with them should begin with a smile. A smile says *'I like you'* and a simple way to make a good impression. Moreover, when a medical representative calls you, say hello in a tone that implies, *'I'm happy to hear from you.'* Never be deceived by first impressions.

Show your genuine interest – It is always better in showing your interest rather than expressing it. *'There is nothing more effective and rewarding than* *showing a genuine interest in other people.'* Moreover, people respond to those who take interest in their welfare. There are many ways of showing interest. For example; learn the names of your medical representatives and pronounce them correctly. The name of the person is the sweetest word he or she likes to hear.

Be natural and affectionate – Whether we're pleasant to be around depends less on the situation than on our behaviour. When you see medical representatives, greet them and express genuine pleasure. When you smile at your medical representatives, the smile must come from your heart. People will respond to a genuine expression of warmth. Never show any superficial interest. Be polite to everyone. *'Being polite doesn't solve anything, but eases everything.'*

Give respect – Everybody deserves respect. Respecting your medical representatives means you value their opinions, feelings and ideas. There are many ways to give respect. For example; treat your medical representatives with courtesy and politeness, encourage them and appreciate the good work. Listen to your medical representatives. Listening is one of the best ways of giving respect to them.

KEY POINTS: How to Deal with Medical Representative?

1. *Lead your medical representatives the way you would like to be led yourself.*
2. *Guide them the way you would like to be guided.*
3. *Give them feedback the way you like to get the feedback.*
4. *Everything you do or say will raise or lower the self-esteem of your medical representative and ultimately affect their performance.*
5. *Treat your medical representatives like colleagues and don't condescend, dictate or berate.*

SUPERVISION

> ***'Supervision is a forum for reflecting on work in the presence of another or others who facilitate that process.'***
>
> ***– Dr. Mike Carroll***

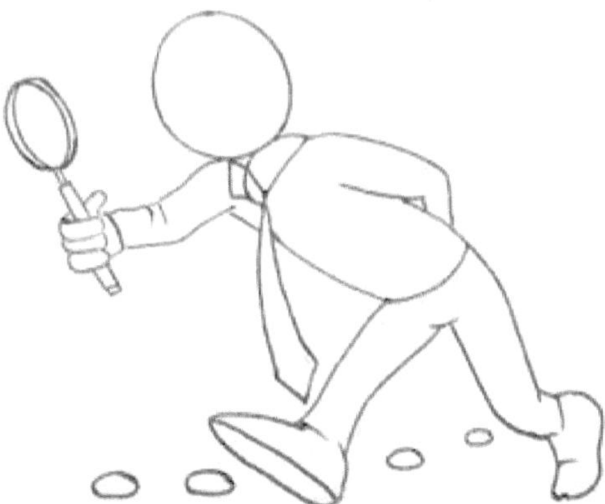

'Vision' implies seeing; the word *'supervision'* can be read as overseeing. A "supervisor" is a person who directs and is responsible for the work of others. The term *'supervisor'* typically refers to one's immediate superior. For example; medical representative's supervisor typically would be the first-line leader. For a First-line leader, supervision is a process of overseeing and managing the day-to- day activities of his medical representatives. This means the process of watching and directing what medical representative does or how something is done. The supervision and guidance of first-line leader encourages medical representatives to be more disciplined in their activities. The supervisions of a first-line leader often include:

Daily call plan – This is a very important tool to monitor the daily activities of a medical representative. The daily work plan gives the direction for a day's work and reduces unplanned working. It also reduces the number of missed calls. Daily work plans can be correlated with the daily reports to verify compliance.

Input utilization - This is another aspect of medical representative's activities that requires constant monitoring. Promotional inputs such as literatures, samples, or gifts are the tools to support the promotion of a given product to doctors. They are to be utilized reasonably in a financially savvy way so as to generate desired prescriptions and achieve territory targets.

Coverage - Medical representatives are expected to meet not less than 95 % of the doctors in the MSL, including repeat visits, in each month. First-line leaders must ensure that the medical representative covers all the doctors (also the chemists). This can be monitored either through formats or through the reporting systems.

> ***It is impossible to be a good leader without being a good supervisor. Developing and maintaining effectiveness as a supervisor is foundational to become a leader.***

MANAGERIAL FUNCTIONS

'Leadership is the ability to get extraordinary achievement from ordinary people'

A leader wears many hats. Effective leadership is about bringing out the best in the people. As a first-line leader your primary responsibility is to ensure that your medical representatives achieve their tasks. The most important task is to achieve their sales objectives on monthly, quarterly and annual basis. To achieve the sales objectives; you need to perform following managerial functions:

1. On the Job Training

> ***No medical representatives are perfect and there is no tailor-made medical representative; hence they need to be trained.***

Training can be defined as 'acquisition of skills and knowledge to perform a current job.' On the job training is the most important function of a first-line leader to train medical representatives for their job. On the job training involves turning work situations into learning opportunities. It is a practical method of the training in which the medical representatives get actual experience by working with their leaders on the job.

First-line leader imparts on the job training to increase personal commitment of medical representatives towards the company and its goal. On the job training has a lot of benefits in the workplace. Joint field work is the important platform for on the job training. The areas of on the job training often include:

- Communications (detailing and retailing)
- Product knowledge
- Presentation skills and Selling skills
- Emotional Intelligence
- Body language

Before giving training, it is essential to find out the strengths as well as areas of improvement of your medical representatives.

2. Planning

> ***Planning is deciding in advance - what to do, when to do and how to do it. It bridges the gap mentally from where we are and where we want to be.***

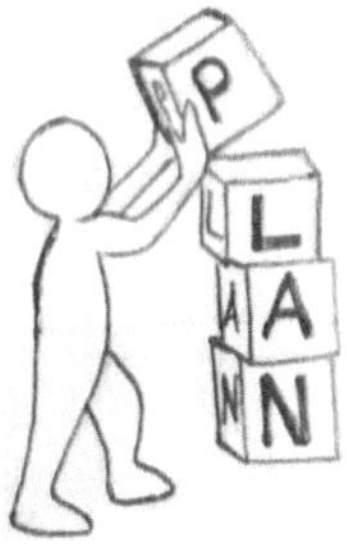

Planning is a process of bridging the gap mentally from where you and your team are now to where you want to be at some future moment regarding accomplishing objectives. This involves setting objectives and developing a strategy to achieve those objectives. Planning provides direction to the medical representatives in order to achieve goals and accomplish objectives. For example; while planning sales for any territory the systematic planning will be based on the followings:

- What is the current base?
- What is the sale you expect from the territory?

- When do you want your medical representative to achieve it?

> ***'Every minute spent in planning saves 10 minutes in execution.'***

3. Organising

> ***'Organising is what you do before you do something, so that when you do it, it is not all mix up.'***
>
> ***– A.A. Milne***

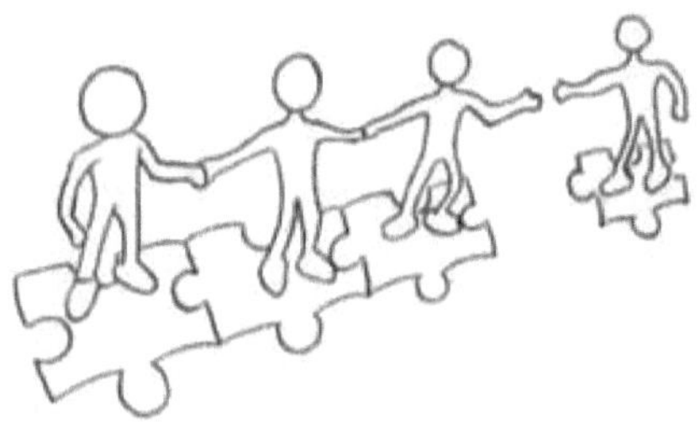

The next step of planning is organizing. Organizing, often called systematic planning, is a process of arranging various steps of planning into a working order. It enables leaders to organize the various steps of planning accordin to their order of priority. Here the first-line leader gives directions and support to the medical representatives so that they will be enthusiastic about exerting effort to execute plans as well as to attain organizational goals. Effective organizing ensures that the right resources are available at the right time, timely execution of the plans and maximizing efficiency.

To become an effective leader, you must be able to organize your own work.

4. Execution

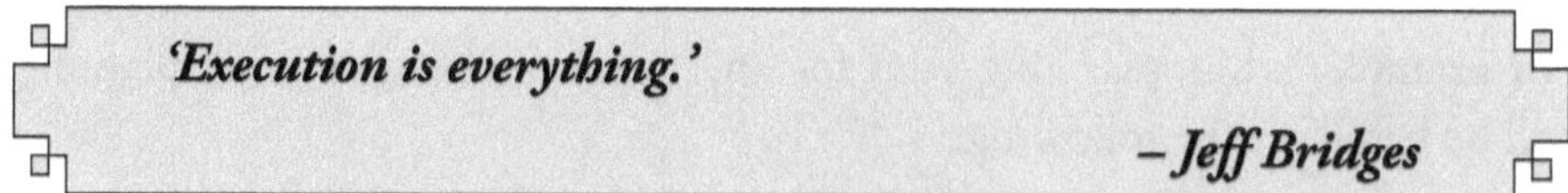

> ***'Execution is everything.'***
>
> ***– Jeff Bridges***

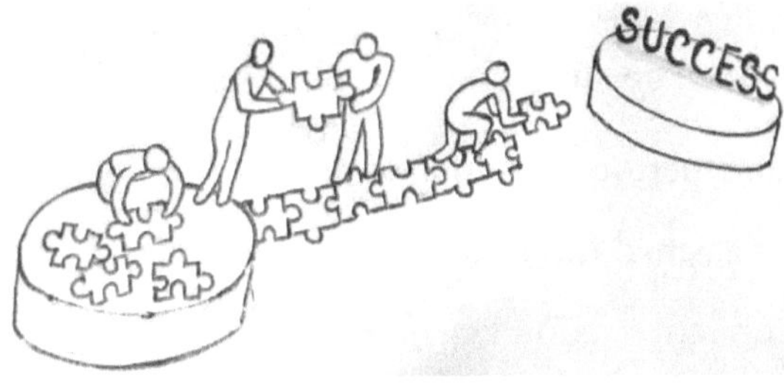

This is the most important function as it transforms strategies and plans into actions. Execution is an ongoing process, not a one-time event. Effective execution has a direct impact on business success and also enhances the reputation and credibility of an organization. First-line leaders are implementers; the ability to execute is one of the most important skills a first-line leader can possess. As a first-line leader, you need to keep your medical representatives motivated to execute the plans.

5. Controlling

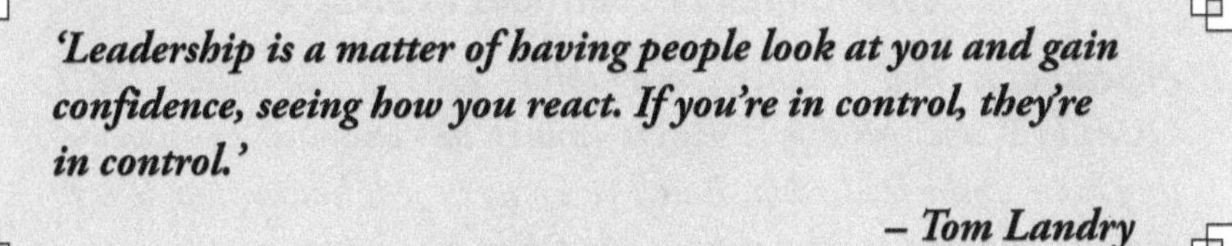

'Leadership is a matter of having people look at you and gain confidence, seeing how you react. If you're in control, they're in control.'

– Tom Landry

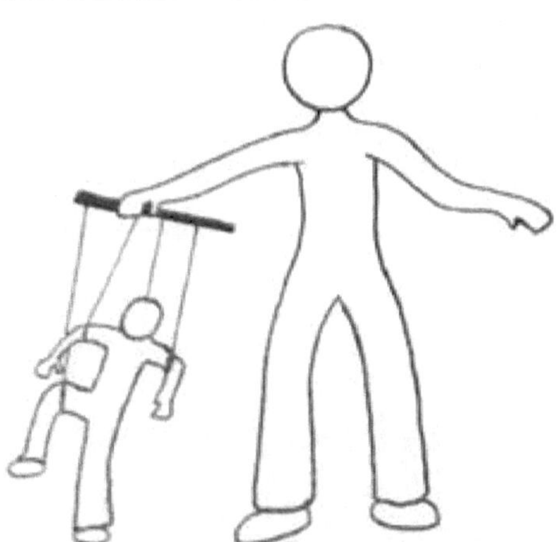

'Controlling involves more than simply being firmly in charge.' Controlling is the final function of the leader which ensures that the execution leads to the desired result, i.e. the performance does not deviate from standards. It is the

process of evaluating the execution and taking corrective measures to ensure that the organizational goal is achieved. Controlling consists of followings:

- Establishing performance standards
- Comparing actual execution against standards
- Taking corrective action when necessary

'Planning and organizing are management functions that ensure efficiency. Execution and Controlling are functions that ensure effectiveness. Efficiency combined with effectiveness leads to excellence in management.'

> ***'Efficiency is the foundation for survival. Effectiveness is the foundation for success.'***
>
> ***– John C. Maxwell***

People cannot be controlled or managed

According to Bob David's, three things can be controlled, TIME, QUALITY and MONEY. People cannot be controlled or managed; they come under leadership. People can only be led; leading people is the opposite of trying to control them. As a first-line leader, power comes to you only when your medical representatives give you their support. When that support comes to you, that is power. Medical representatives give you that power and watch your behaviour. If you deflect that power back to them, they begin to trust you and give you more support.

'Give power, don't take it. Power enables control. Control engages. Feeling controlled disengages.'

FIRST-LINE LEADER IS AN IMPORTANT POSITION

First-line leaders are the most important position in a Pharmaceutical company. They are the key to any successful operation. They can change the scenario completely. Today the role of a first-line leader has changed in view of the changed environment. The variety of tasks undertaken in the role makes it interesting and challenging. Despite the challenges, this is a job that often gives great satisfaction and can be immensely enjoyable. **Vivek Hattangadi** has mentioned in his book **"Pharma First- Line Leader To CEO"** that a first-line leader performs various roles which make the position interesting and challenging. For example:

Coaching

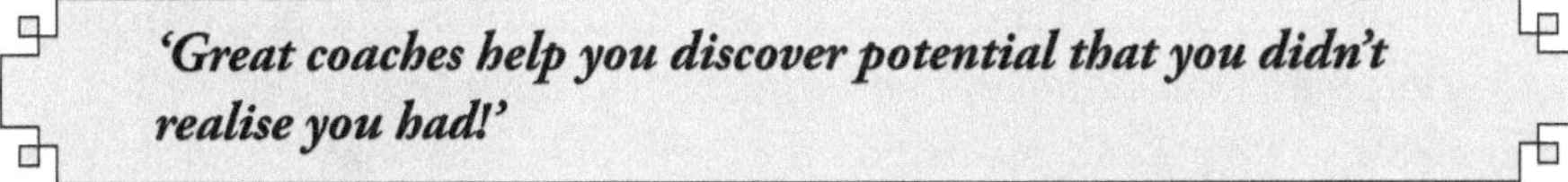

'Great coaches help you discover potential that you didn't realise you had!'

The role of a good coach is to turn a group of people into a committed team where each person is a star performer.' Coaching is probably one of the most delightful aspects of a leader's job because it focuses on the growth and success of people. Coaching is the way of encouraging and supporting medical representatives to develop their existing skills and to achieve goals. Coaching can be done before, during or after the joint field work with medical representatives. During coaching, the first-line leader makes corrections, gives advice, fine tunes and hones the performance. The intent is to provide specific expertise and focus and to stimulate achievements.

HRD Manager

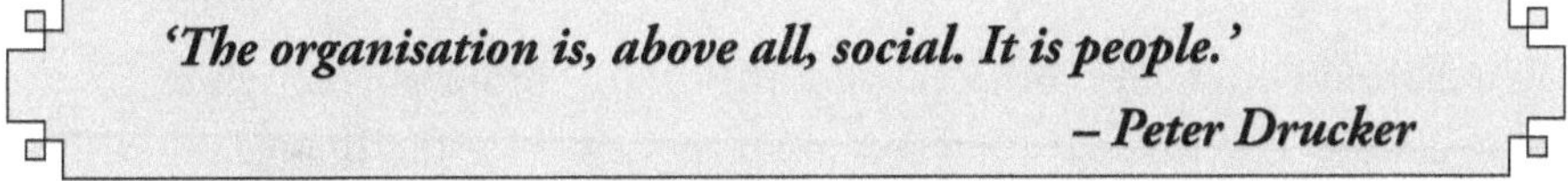

'The organisation is, above all, social. It is people.'
– Peter Drucker

Employee retention has emerged as the workplace issue of the decade. The success of an organisation is determined by its ability to retain its people. The most important job of an HRD manager is retention of people. Employee retention refers to the various processes which let the employees remain in the organisation for a longer period of time. Retention of people is a financial gain for the organization. First-line leaders also play the role of an HRD manager. They retain people, identifying the right people for the job and also maintaining a data bank of potential people for the future. Always retain the right people, but for those medical representatives, whose integrity is in question, immediately bring it to the notice of your superior. To be successful, you should have zero tolerance for dishonest or corrupt people.

Brand Manager

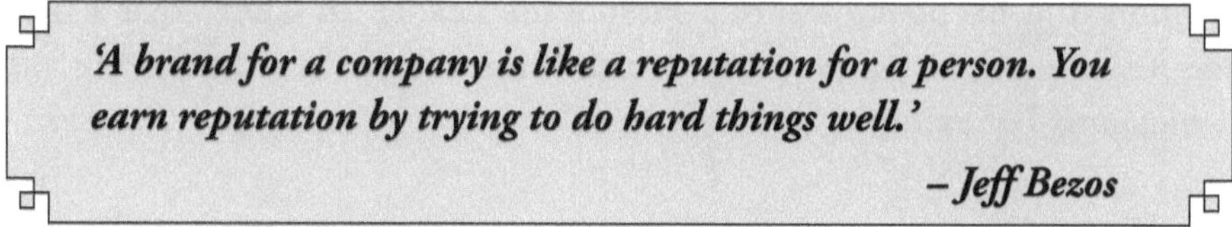

> ***'A brand for a company is like a reputation for a person. You earn reputation by trying to do hard things well.'***
>
> ***– Jeff Bezos***

The brands are the important assets for an organisation. The brand manager is a person who plans, develops and directs marketing efforts for the brands. They create strategies and ensure that the brands resonate with the current and potential prescribers. Building a brand is nothing but generating prescriptions through successful implementation of strategies. First-line leaders are the strategy implementers. They also ensure that the prescription shares of the brands are increased by getting the strategies implemented by the medical representatives. In addition, they can give market feedback on competitor activities to PMT. Thus they can help PMT to design better strategies to beat the competition.

Finance Manager

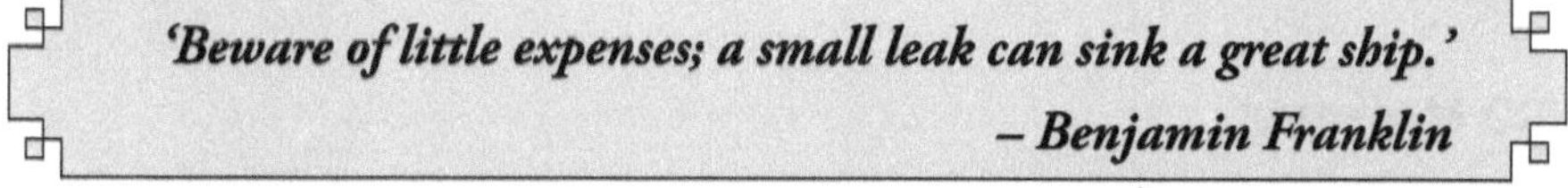

> ***'Beware of little expenses; a small leak can sink a great ship.'***
>
> ***– Benjamin Franklin***

Financial activities are complex and the most important activities of the organisation. The finance managers are responsible for the financial health of an organisation and their actions directly affect the profitability. Profitability is essential for survival of any organisation. First-line leaders play the role of a finance manager by optimising the limited resources for better output. Promotional inputs like physician's samples, gifts and LBLs are investments and they have to ensure expected return on these investments.

CRM Manager

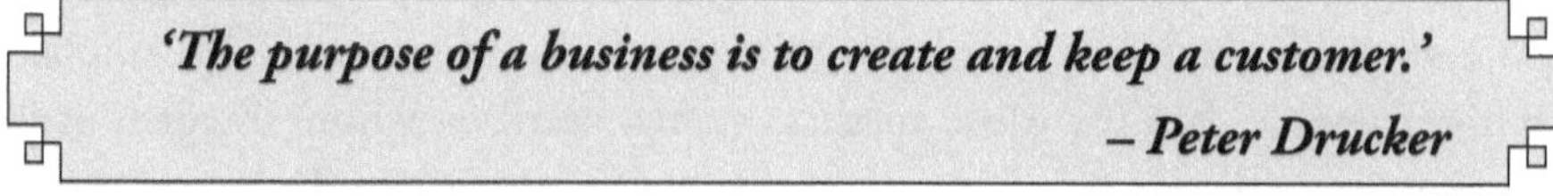

> ***'The purpose of a business is to create and keep a customer.'***
>
> ***– Peter Drucker***

CRM or Customer Relationship Management is a business approach that seeks to create, develop and enhance relationships with targeted doctors in order to improve customer value and corporate profitability. The objective of

CRM is to look after your potential doctors so that they keep on prescribing your product. First-line leaders can play the role of a CRM manager as they have direct contact with the doctors. They need to build trust and confidence among them. They supposed to do healthy CRM which upgrades the quality of prescriptions, which leads to a strong brand.

Chapter 2

COMPETENCES OF A FIRST-LINE LEADER

'The success of leadership depends on competence.'

'The future belongs to the competent. Get good, get better, be the best.'

Competence of an individual is the ability to do something successfully or efficiently. Leadership behaviours as well as skills which contribute to superior performance are known as the leadership competencies. However, the competences needed for a particular position may change depending on the specific leadership level in the organisation.

First-line leders need certain prerequisites. They must have certain core competencies like emotional intelligence, decisiveness, team building, time management etc.

1. EMOTIONAL INTELLIGENCE

Emotion is a signal of information and people follow these signals. Effective leaders have the ability to manage their emotions brilliantly and so are able to produce results even in high pressure situations. This ability is known as Emotional Intelligence or EI. EI gives leaders a variety of attributes, such as the ability to manage relationships, influence and inspire others. The term emotional intelligence was popularised in 1995 by psychologist Daniel Goleman in his first book, **'Emotional Intelligence.'** Daniel Goleman described emotional intelligence as a person's ability to manage his/her feelings so that those feelings are expressed appropriately and effectively. According to Goleman, emotional intelligence is the biggest single indicator of success in the workplace. In fact, EI has become a necessity for all of us. The significance of emotional intelligence increases, the higher you go in the organisation.

EI is not the opposite of logical intelligence which is conventionally known as intelligence or IQ. IQ convinces people by facts whereas EQ convinces by reasoning. In pharmaceutical selling, where there are many brands with the same molecule, trying to convince a doctor with facts and logic may not work, whereas you may be able to convince through emotional appeal. IQ is necessary, but it is not enough to become a great leader. Leadership requires more of EQ than IQ.

Emotional Intelligence is a key to successful leadership. The success of a leader depends on the ability to read other people's emotions and then react appropriately to them. The leader with strong leadership quality also tends to be more emotionally intelligent. Emotional intelligence helps leader to manage his emotions as well as others with empathy.

> ***'Emotional intelligence is not something that can be developed by sitting and reading instruction manuals. It needs practice.'***

Components of Emotional Intelligence

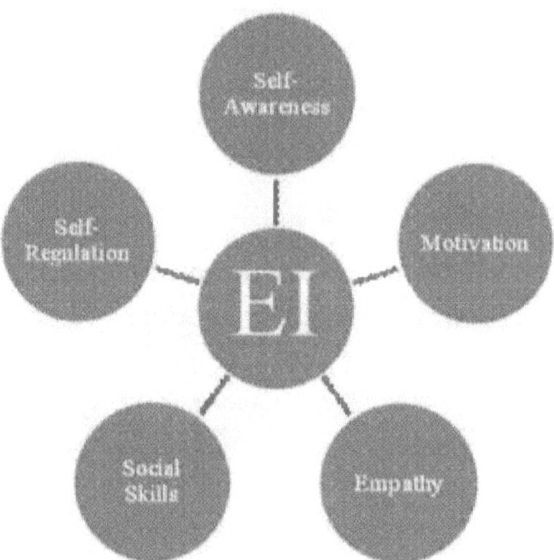

As stated by Daniel Goleman, there are five components of emotional intelligence that enable the leader to maximise their own and their team's performance. These five components are divided into two groups:

1	**Personal Competence**	The way you manage yourselves	Ability to be aware of and manage your emotions; it focuses more on you individually than your interactions with others. It comprised of 'Self-awareness,' 'Self-regulation' and 'Self- motivation'
2	**Social Competence**	The way you handle relationship	Ability to understand people's moods, behaviours, and motives. It comprised of 'Social awareness' and 'Social skills'

Self-awareness: This is the first component of emotional intelligence and refers to the ability to understand your own emotions. Self-awareness also means having a clear understanding of the effect of your own actions, moods, and emotions on other people. To improve your self-awareness, you must be capable of monitoring your own emotions, recognising different emotional reactions, and then correctly identifying each particular emotion.

Self-regulation: This is nothing but expressing your emotions appropriately. In addition to being aware of your own emotions, you need to regulate and manage your emotions. Self-regulations are very important for a leader. Leaders who are in control of their feelings and impulses can create environment of trust and fairness. First-line leaders who are skilled in self-regulation tend to be flexible in their approach and adapt well to change.

Self-motivations: This plays a key role in emotional intelligence. Emotionally intelligent leaders are internally motivated because they have a passion to fulfil their own inner needs and goals. First-line leaders who are competent in this area tend to be action-oriented. They set goals, have a high need for achievement, and are always looking for ways to do better. They also tend to be very committed and are good at taking the initiative when a task is put forth before them.

Social awareness: This is often called empathy and is the ability to understand how others are feeling, i.e. *'feeling as someone.'* This involves more than just being able to recognise the emotional states of others. This is a critical skill for first-line leaders, who work closely to inspire and motivate medical representatives. Empathetic leaders are perceptive of others emotions and take an active interest in their concerns. Social awareness or empathy is the most important component of EI.

Social skills: This is the ability to interact well with others, and an important aspect of emotional intelligence. Social skill is the culmination of the other components of emotional intelligence. Social skills are the key for success of a leader because the leader's task is to get work done through other people and social skill makes that possible. In a professional setting, this skill helps first-line leader to build relationships with medical representatives. Social skills mean relationship management which involves active listening, leadership skills and persuasiveness. Social skills allow leaders to put their emotional intelligence into work.

KEY POINTS: Emotional Intelligence

1. *Difficult situations can interfere with productivity, impact upon physical and emotional health, and generally cause medical representatives to underperform. First-line leaders with high EI can deal with difficult situations powerfully.*
2. *As a first-line leader, the quality of your life will depend on the way you handle pressure. High EI helps you to handle pressure.*
3. *Emotional intelligence is a choice and a set of skills you need to build every day.*

2. DECISIVENESS

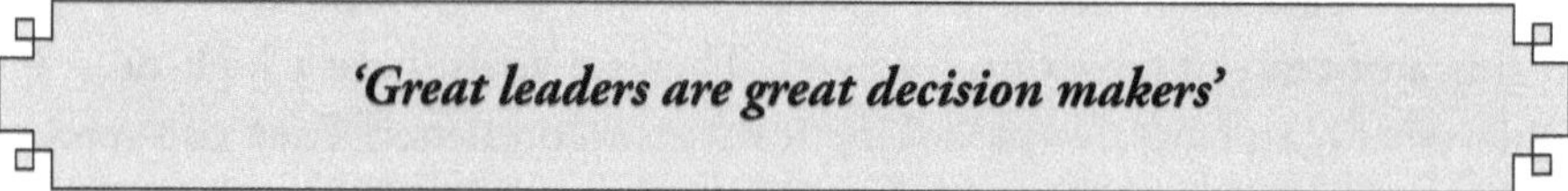
'Great leaders are great decision makers'

In each leadership role, it is necessary for leaders to make decisions. The decision-making is the process of choosing between two or more courses of action. Decisiveness is the ability to analyse a situation and make a right decision on time. Decision-making is part of a leader's daily expectations and is a core of managerial competence. Not taking decision is also a decision. In fact, a leader or a manager is primarily a decision maker. Decision-making can be hard as there is considerable risk involved while making important and critical decisions. Almost any decision involves some conflicts or dissatisfaction. The success or failures of a leader depends on the ability to make right decisions and implement them effectively. Decisive first-line leaders gain respect from their medical representatives.

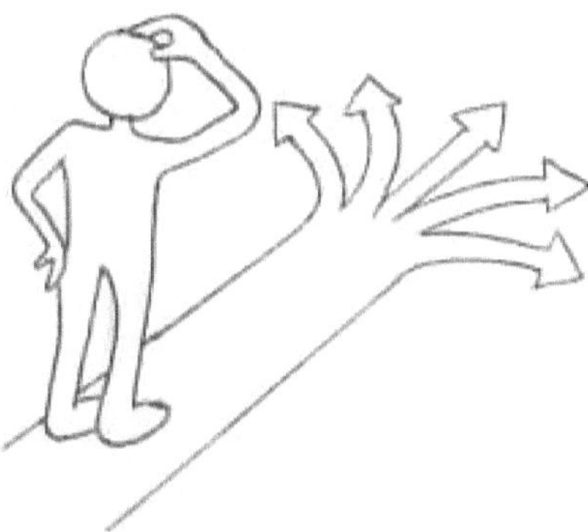

> ***'Leaders do not always make right decisions, but they make their decisions right'***

As a first-line leader, it is likely that you spend time with your medical representatives all day every day. When making a decision, think about the effect your decision will have on the job aspect of your medical representatives, but not strictly on whether or not it will make them like you more. The decision-making process involves several steps. The following five steps can help you in better decision-making:

1. **Define the problem:** A problem is defined as a discrepancy between an existing and desired state of affairs. The decision- making process begins when you identify the real problem. If the problem is not precisely defined, then it will affect every step of the decision-making process.

2. **Gather information:** The need for a decision arises because a leader is faced with a problem and alternative courses of action are available. In deciding which option to choose you will need all the information which is relevant to your decision; and you must have some criteria on the basis of which you can choose the best alternative.

3. **Develop appropriate option:** At this stage, creative thinking is required. You need to open your mind into wide focus to consider all

possible options and then to sort out the appropriate option from the number of possible options. Appropriate means capable of being done

4. **Implementation:** After the decision is made, you need to discuss with medical representatives about the implementation. A detailed implementation plan ensures proficiency in the decisional process.
5. **Review your decision:** Reviewing your decision is a part of the overall decision-making process. This is an important step for further development of your decision-making skills. In this step, consider the result of your decision and evaluate whether or not it has resolved the problem you identified in step 1. If the decision has not resolved the problem, repeat the steps to make a new decision.

However, a leader often has to make quick decisions without enough time to systematically go through the above steps. In such situations the most effective decision-making strategy is to keep an eye on your goals and then let your gut feeling suggest you make the right choice.

KEY POINTS: Decisiveness

1. *Do not decide without complete information.*
2. *Avoid making decisions under the influence and prejudices.*
3. *Don't over trust the opinion of your team members.*
4. *Don't decide in hurry and also don't postpone taking important decisions.*
5. *Have some flexibility in plan of action.*

The ability of a leader to make right decisions on time develops with practice, and this is possible only when the leader acts in harmony with the circumstances and the situation.

'The ability to make a decision and stick to it is the cornerstone of good leadership skills.'

3. TEAM BUILDING

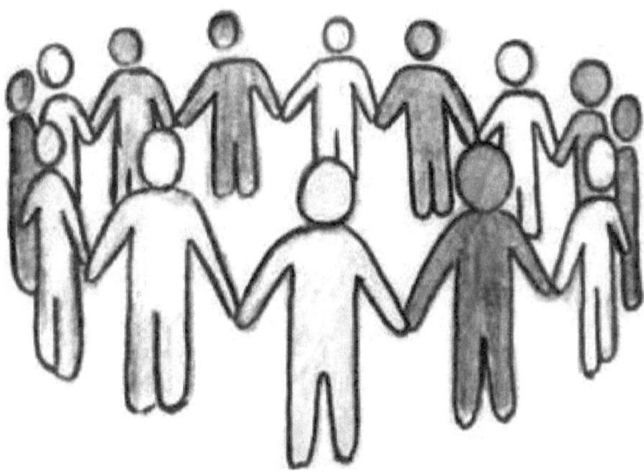

A team is a group of two or more people working together towards a common goal; whereas, when two or more people are classed together, it is known as a group. A team is like a car which consists of multiple parts joined together to accomplish a particular task whereas an example of a group is *'a group of people waiting at a bus stop.'* A team differentiates itself from a group on various dimensions. All teams are a group, but a group is not necessarily a team.

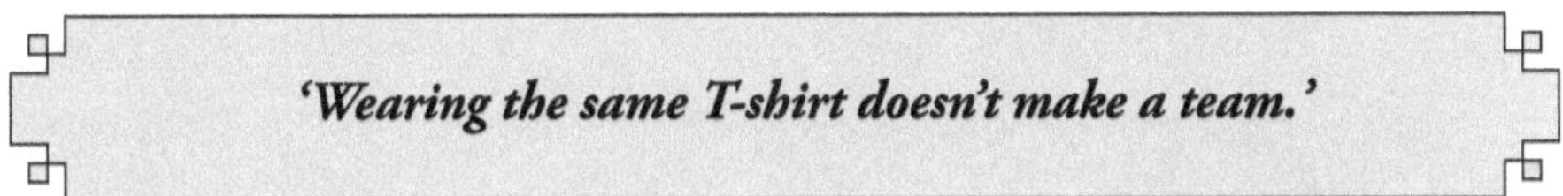

'Wearing the same T-shirt doesn't make a team.'

The basic difference is, in a group members are independent but in a team members are interdependent. The feature of a good team is *'the whole is greater than the sum of its parts.'* This means that the ability of a team is much greater than the skills of its members put together. In the team, members believe that as part of a team, everything that they do or don't do, impacts team performance, hence they make sure that no matter whose job it is, it must be done. The success of a team is dependent upon every member within the team and to achieve success, the leader needs to ensure that they come together, keep together and work together.

> ***'Coming together is a beginning, staying together is progress, and working together is success.'***
>
> ***– Henry Ford***

A pharmaceutical organisation cannot be effective without teamwork. Teamwork is the key to increase productivity and profitability. In our context, teamwork is something that is nurtured and developed with a cooperative effort between the medical representatives and first-line leaders. Teamwork benefits everyone in the group as well as leader. The keys to effective team work include recognising and managing the team's dynamics, communicating effectively and encouraging collaboration, and managing conflicts and other problems that arise.

Teamwork Lessons from Birds Flying in V Formation

Most of you have looked up in the sky and noticed a flock of migrating birds flying in V formation. This is one of the best examples of teamwork.

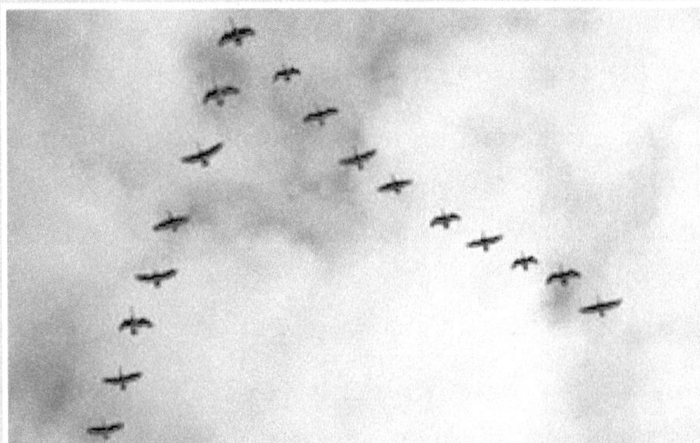

By flying in V formation, each bird provides additional lift and reduces air resistance for the birds flying behind it. It has estimated that by doing so, the whole flock adds 71% greater flying range than if each bird flew alone.

Each bird keeps its place behind the leader. When the leader gets tired, it drops back and another bird moves to the leadership position. This change in position happens many times which offers everyone the opportunity to serve as a leader as well as a follower.

They also frequently make loud honking sounds as they fly together. Similarly, when working on teams, it is exceedingly important for each team member to communicate regularly with all the other team members.

'Team work divides the work and multiplies the success.'

– Khushboo A. Gala

Role of First-Line Leaders in Team Building

Team building is the most important, the first activity, the first-line leader has to do in order to drive medical representatives in right direction and bring the best out of them. Team building is a collective term for various types of activities where the leader acts as a facilitator. Below are the important roles of a first-line leader in team building.

Develop trust: Trust is defined as *'the inner sense of acceptance you have of others with whom you are able to share secrets, knowing they are safe. The sense that things are fine, that nothing can disrupt the bond between you and the other.'* For a leader to work as a team, building trust is very important. Long-term relationships are built on the foundation of trust. In fact, trust and leadership go hand in hand. Trust takes long time to build, but can be destroyed instantly.

Trustworthy leaders extract better output. When you trust your medical representatives, they will feel confident and work with better productivity, loyalty and high morale. When medical representatives place their trust in their leaders, it is with conviction that they further act, that they would be able to accomplish tasks set before them.

Create a vision – You have to share your vision with your medical representatives and inspire them to support that vision. Only you can do it. Create an inspiring vision. Provide the big picture and keep the vision of the big picture before yourself and your medical representatives. Every team member has a role to play, and every role has its part in contributing to the bigger picture.

Be loyal – Loyalty is a highly valued character trait desired between the first-line leader and medical representatives. Loyalty is the glue that holds relationships together. You can create loyalty through your words and actions.

Make the work enjoyable – Always create an enjoyable work environment. Encourage entrepreneurial activity like risk-taking, i.e. allow your medical representatives to be entrepreneurial and to test their ideas.

Avoid micromanagement – Avoid close supervision; do not over boss; do not dictate. Work hard on those delegation skills and learn to trust your team to develop and deliver. Intervene when necessary to aid the team in resolving issues.

4. TIME MANAGEMENT

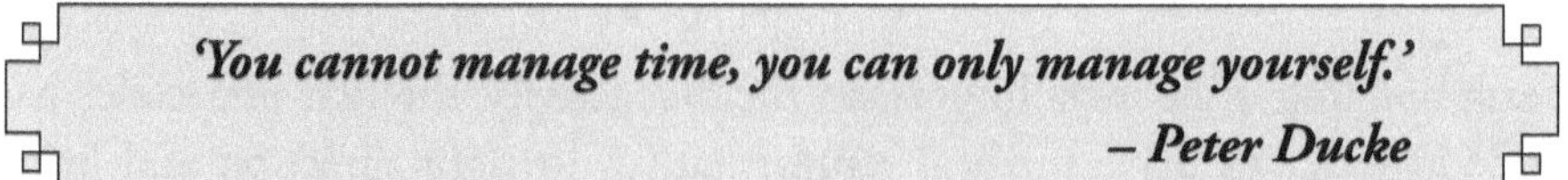

'You cannot manage time, you can only manage yourself.'
– Peter Ducke

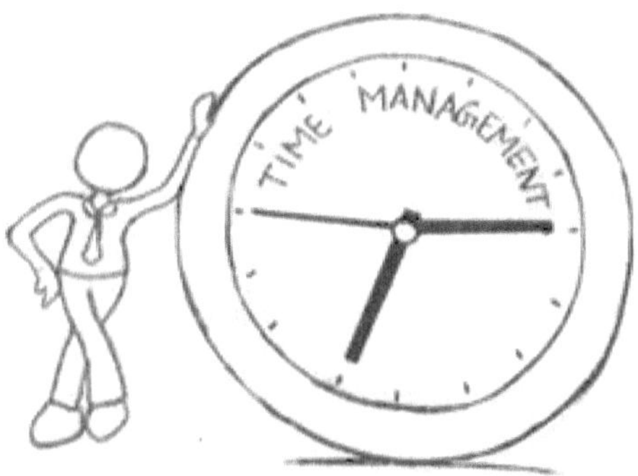

Time is defined as a finite period or interval between two successive events. Time never halts for any one, once wasted, it can never be regained. Time is very precious; it has to be put to the best use of it.

Every activity requires time. Time management is the process of organising and planning how to divide your time between specific activities. Effective time management will enable you to complete more assignments in shorter time frames. Time management can also be termed as life management because time management is a core discipline that determines the quality of your life.

No one in this world is born with a good time manager. To become a good time manager, you need to learn about it. It cannot be learned overnight; it requires persistent effort over a long time. Proper time management ensures greater productivity and personal fulfilment.

Effective management of time requires careful consideration of following factors:

To do list – A 'to do list' is the only work which you definitely have to do. Preparing a 'to do list' is the most important area for managing time. Before you can manage your time, you need to have a list of things, what you do, i.e. it must be visible. The lack of visibility can lead to different problems. For example:

- You may forget to do it.
- There may be delay.
- There are possibilities, that you are doing things which are not important.

- You may miss out important tasks and so on.

Preparing a 'to do list' is simple and is the first step of managing time.

KEY POINTS: To Do List

1. *It will ensure that you won't forget them.*
2. *You can keep yourself on track.*
3. *To do list will increase your commitment to them.*

Apply common sense – There are many activities necessary to live a normal life; and time is divided between these activities according to the need. It is crucial that you must periodically evaluate your own use of time. Good time management principles are universal and basic common sense. If you apply common sense, then you will be a long way down the road to improving your time management. For example:

- Block out a regular time every day for dealing with routine work.
- Mobiles are great time wasters. Because of the added features, more time is being used on the mobiles. Control your use of mobiles and also try to switch it off when you need some quiet time to concentrate on something.
- Focus on doing only one task at a time.
- You need to be disciplined in keeping important items at home and at the workplace. However, misplaced items result in a lot of wasted time and effort.

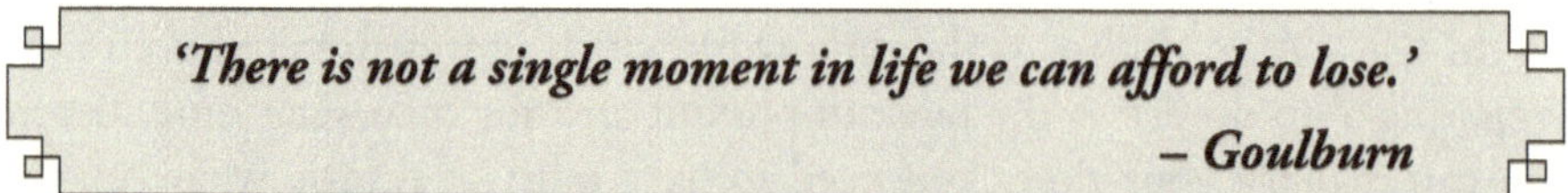

'There is not a single moment in life we can afford to lose.'
– Goulburn

Control procrastination – This is the biggest challenge of time management. Procrastination is the opposite of actions which means unnecessary delaying work, that to without any reason. As the proverb says, *'Procrastination is the thief of time,'* and it destroys initiative. For effective time management and to become successful, first try to get rid of habits of procrastination because you cannot escape the responsibility of tomorrow by avoiding it today. Followings are some of the ways to overcome procrastination:

- The first step to overcome procrastination is to recognise it.
- Keep a note of all cut off dates of sending formats; feedbacks etc.
- Prioritise your things to do as per the importance.
- If you have a large task to do, then break it down into smaller parts and deal with those smaller parts one at a time.
- Nothing will work unless you do and do it now. A thousand mile journey begins with a single step. Take the step and leave inertia behind.
- Let time be your servant rather than your master.
- Never leave till tomorrow, which you can finish today

> ***'When there is a hill to climb, don't think that waiting will make it smaller.'***

Say 'No' assertively –There is a saying, *'I don't know the key to success, but the key to failure is trying to please everybody.'* One of the challenges people face is their inability to say 'no' to the request of others. An understanding of assertiveness will help you say 'no' in a way leaving others without the feeling of guilt. You have to say 'no' to those people and activities that aren't aligned with your most important goals. An assertive individual will have a better time implementing and maintaining good time management routines.

KEY POINTS: How to Say 'No'

1. *Say 'No' politely and diplomatically and most importantly don't delay in saying it.*
2. *Always say it with a reason.*
3. *Always suggest an alternative to the 'No.'*

> ***The art of leadership is saying 'no' not 'yes.' It is very easy to say yes.***
>
> ***– Tony Blair***

*"Time management refers to **Effective Working** and not **Fast Working**"*

CASE STUDY

Debasish is working as an area sales manager in Xenom Pharmaceuticals Ltd. a top Indian multinational company. He is always very busy with his work, making calls, meeting KOLs, attending CMEs and many more activities. He does not find time for his family. Taking care of his family is the most important goal in his life, but he is unable to fulfill it because he is busy with many different activities. These activities are taking him away from his goal. His performance at work goes down. His family life is in a wreck.

What should he do? On priority, he should learn to know his priorities.

Prioritization is putting things in order of importance. To be able to prioritize your goals, you should first say 'NO' to procrastination and then decide which goal you should focus upon first. For effective prioritization, it is very crucial to differentiate things as urgent and important. It also helps to reduce stress.

Over 85% of your time should be spent on important things before they become urgent and reach a fire-fighting situation. Here for instance, Debashish should have spent every Sunday / holiday with his family.

He could have taken a two-week vacation with his family. This creates the upward spiral of growth. Spending quality time could have lifted him to a new level. Debashish should not have procrastinated taking holidays.

He could have maintained a quality work-life balance which could have increased his performance at work.

Lesson: Achieving work-life balance should be a priority for anyone – more so as you climb up the career ladder.

'The key is not prioritisze what's on your schedule, but to schedule your priorities'

– Stephen R. Covey

Prioritise your task: Stephen Covey's Time Management Matrix

For proper time management, you need to learn how to utilise your time effectively by doing more important tasks in the time you have and also learn to put aside the less important tasks. To be successful as a leader, you must work on the basis of priority. The Stephen Covey's time management matrix is an effective method of organising your priorities. It differentiates between activities that are important and those that are urgent.

- **Important** activities have an outcome that leads to the achievement of your goals.
- **Urgent** activities demand immediate attention.

Stephen Covey's approach to time management is to create time to focus on important things before they become urgent. Once you learn the basic principles of organising your activities according to the principles of this tool, you will likely be able to eliminate a number of time wasting activities and unproductive behaviours. Stephen Covey's tools are designed to maximise your productivity and eliminate unnecessary or irrelevant activities through a 4-quadrant system.

Quad 1	**Quad 2**
URGENT AND IMPORTANT **It's a necessity** **Example:** *Crisis* *Deadline-driven activities*	**IMPORTANT BUT NOT URGENT** **Need to Focus** **Example:** *Preparation and planning Relationship-building*
Quad 3	**Quad 4**
URGENT BUT NOT IMPORTANT **To be minimised or** delegated **Example:** *Meeting other people's priorities* *Frequent interruptions*	**NON-IMPORTANT AND NON-URGENT** **To be avoided** **Example:** *Playing with mobile* *Junk mail*

The four quadrants of the time management matrix reflect four different types of activities: Important and Urgent, Important and Non-Urgent, Non-important and Urgent, Non-important and Non-urgent.

Quadrant 1: We have important and urgent things that require maximum attention and need to be dealt with immediately. Perhaps spending too much time in this quadrant will lead to stress and you will be caught in a never-ending cycle of crisis management and firefighting. There are many important and non-urgent activities that become urgent and important through procrastination, lack of planning etc.

Quadrant 2: We have important but not urgent things that do not require your immediate attention, and need to be planned for. These are our priorities and goals. As a first-line leader, you should spend most of your time in this quadrant for long term achievement of goals. Here you have to take initiative to act on. You can get more time to spend here by avoiding Quad 4 activities. Ignoring Quad 2 activities enlarges Quad 1, creating stress and burnout.

Quadrant 3: We have urgent but unimportant things, which should be minimised or eliminated. If they are important at all, they are important to someone else. We spend a lot of time in Quad 3, meeting other people's priorities and expectations, while thinking we are really in Quad 1.

Quadrant 4: We have unimportant and also not urgent things, which means the time waster which must be avoided.

Quadrant 1: DO, don't wait.

Quadrant 2: FOCUS, keep your maximum time.

Quadrant 3: DELEGATE, don't add burden of these tasks.

Quadrant 4: DUMP, avoid it.

When you do well your high priority task, you will make an enormous and significant contribution.

'Successful leaders prioritise their tasks and assignments according their importance.'

SITUATION

When Territory Becomes Vacant

Vacant territories can weaken a pharmaceutical organisation. Generally, no territory should be vacant. However, vacant territories are created by the natural attritions and repositioning of medical representatives. There are different reasons for attrition. Moreover, in the current scenario jobs are freely available with an increased number of companies as well as the number of divisions. You have to maintain the sale of vacant territories. In order to do that you have to ensure the followings:

1. *Coverage of all the prescribers or the VIP doctors regularly till the vacancy filled up. Try to visit them independently, if not possible then with any of your team members from your rest of the territories.*
2. *For pool territories, ensure the coverage by other team members of the same territory. Be in touch with the important doctors of the vacant territory over phone or through whatsapp, sms.*
3. *Be in constant touch with your stockist and important chemist of the vacant territory.*
4. *Be proactive, you should be on the constant lookout for good prospective candidates in each territory.*
5. *Once you find suitable candidates who can match the qualifying criteria of your organisation, you should take a formal interview of these candidates and recommend them to your superiors for next round of interviews.*

7 HABITS OF FIRST–LINE LEADERS

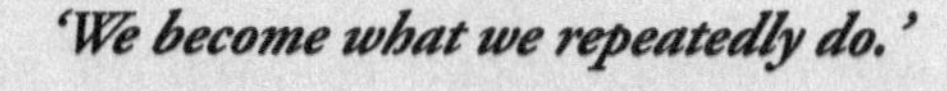
'We become what we repeatedly do.'

Whatever we do repeatedly becomes our habit. A habit is a routine of behaviour that is repeated subconsciously. Habits are powerful factors of our lives. According to Stephen R. Covey, *'Habit is the intersection of Knowledge, Skills and Desires.'* Knowledge is the theoretical paradigm, i.e. *'what to do and the why.'* Skills are *'how to do.'* Desire is the motivation, the *'want to do.'* In order to make something a habit in our lives, we have to have all three. First-line leadership is associated with a lot of choices as well as making decisions. Each decision you make has an effect on your overall character. As you practice making better choices, those choices become habits, and those good habits have the power to transform your leadership. The first-line positions are very important in the hierarchy; they need to practice the following habits:

1. **Result orientation**

   The most important habit of a successful first-line leader is being result oriented. Result orientation is not only 100% achievement on target, it is beyond that. Result orientation is nothing but a mindset that defines achievement despite odds and it is about a high level of ownership for results. Result orientation means having the drive and passion to accomplish goals, excel in all you do, and be successful. Result oriented leaders are always striving to improve their work; they meet deadlines, maintain high standards, and look to overcome any circumstance in a positive manner. They strive to develop their understanding and competence at a task by exerting a high level of effort. They do not give excuses for non-achievement of budgets rather they plan for contingencies and demonstrate a strong desire to achieve against all odds. They are rarely 100% satisfied, and therefore are always looking for ways to improve.

> ***'Be intensely result oriented in everything you do. This is a key characteristic of high performer.'***
>
> ***– Brian Tracy***

2. **Strategy execution**

   Execution is a discipline, and a systematic way of exposing plans and acting on it. Execution of strategies is the main role of a first-line leader. The success of an organisation depends on the execution; however, organisations lose 40 to 60% of their strategies during execution. Successful execution is as much as about establishing and defining your credibility as an effective first-line leader. Successful execution requires a comprehensive understanding of the business process, its people and its environment and the first-line leader is the only person in a position to achieve those understandings. First-line leaders should prepare detailed execution plans for the strategies which involve at a territory level down to a customer wise and brand wise level. They must track execution, review status and revise plans to ensure robust execution.

> ***'Strategy execution is the responsibility that makes or breaks executives.'***
>
> ***– Alan Branche***

3. **Develop analytical skills**

   Analytical skills have become more important than ever. Analytical skills help leaders to adapt to changes in the business environment. Analytical skills or analytical thinking are the ability to collect, analyse information and make decisions. Analytical skills allow you to solve complex problems by making decisions in the most effective way. Analytical skills help to break down larger problems into smaller parts which are easier to solve. For example; analytical skills can be used to convert area and territory budgets into detailed customer wise brand wise plans. First-line leaders should strive to improve their analytical orientation. Developing analytical skills of a leader is very important and it needs practice. Practicing this skill can sharpen your decision-making abilities, enhance problem-solving capabilities, and ultimately drive better outcomes for your medical representatives.

> ***'A lack of analytical skills could keep you from making progress in your career.'***

4. **Develop medical representatives**

   The growth of a pharmaceutical organisation is directly proportional to the growth of the medical representatives. As a leader, you should dedicate time to make sure medical representatives are growing and becoming even better at what they do so that they can be the most productive for you. You should provide effective leadership to your team; coach them on a regular basis. Use joint field work as an opportunity to develop your team member's skills as well as knowledge. If you want to win, you need to help your medical representative win.

> ***'The best minute you spend is the one you invest in people'***
>
> ***– Ken Blanchard***

5. **Doctor sensitivity**

   Doctors are the focus point in pharmaceutical business. They keep our business running. Being sensitive is a caring approach and doctor sensitivity means being aware of a doctor's reactions, moods, needs and wants. You need to pay close attention to your doctor's reaction. You have to develop skills to look within the doctor and find the needs. These needs which doctors may or may not inform you about, you have to get those needs out into the open. *'The result of a business is a satisfied customer'* and that you should anticipate and satisfy the doctor's needs. Doctor sensitivity will give you an opportunity to grow and become even more successful in your career.

> ***This world is a world of competition. 'If we don't care our customers, someone else will'***

6. **Proactive**

   It means more than merely taking initiative. Being proactive means recognising our responsibilities to make things happen. Proactive leaders take responsibility for their management roles by engaging and cooperating with their team, leading by example, and always looking for ways to improve. Their reflexes are like a chess player, wherein they plan their moves three steps ahead. The future belongs to those leaders who see possibilities before they become obvious. They can anticipate the issues as well as have plans to solve them. *'If you want to bring about changes, be Proactive.'*

> ***'The way to bring about change is to be proactive and active.'***
>
> ***– Octavia Spencer***

7. **Striving for excellence**

   Excellence is an important part of professionalism in any job. Excellence is a journey, not a goal. Striving for excellence is an attitude, a belief, a choice, a lifestyle and a trait that virtually every first-line leader should have. Striving for excellence is a sign of quality; you won't always get it but it involves trying to put the best effort into everything you do. Always do your best and you will have nothing to regret. Success doesn't come to those who sit and wait, it is necessary to work towards your vision. Engage with your vision, keep taking actions. Great leaders are never satisfied; they continually strive to be better.

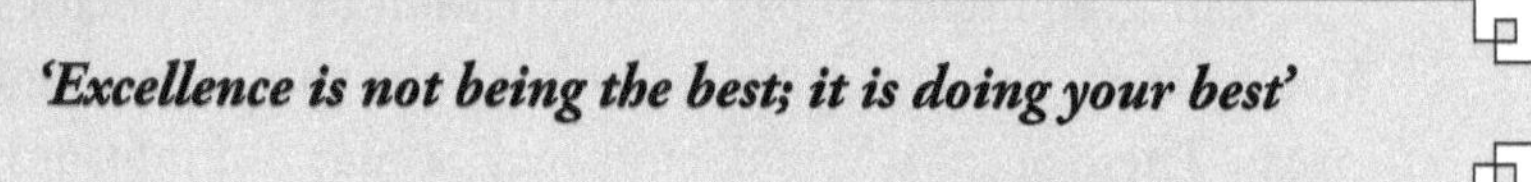

'Excellence is not being the best; it is doing your best'

Chapter 3

JOINT FIELD WORK

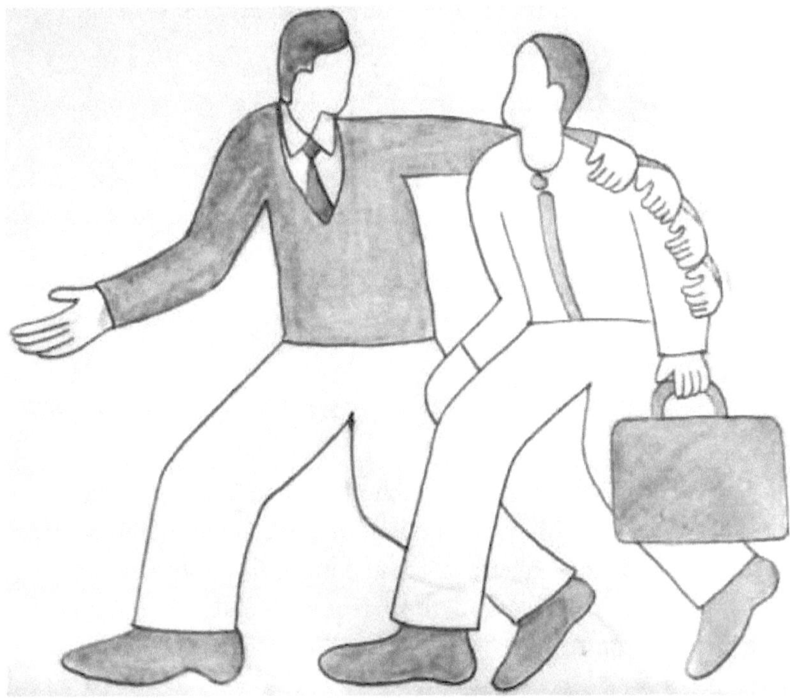

Field visit by leaders along with medical representatives is commonly referred to as joint field work (JFW). During JFW, medical representatives and leaders work jointly, calling on doctors, chemists and stockists. First-line leaders spend 95% of their time in field work. JFW is one of the important sales building steps in which both the leader and the medical representatives work in a spirit of mutuality to enhance brand sales. This is a great opportunity for imparting on the job training to the medical representatives. JFW is also a window of opportunity to observe execution of strategy and use of promotional inputs. In today's scenario, where medical representative's standards are falling, work culture is declining; morals are changing not only in the internal customers but also in the external customers, the joint field work is developing as an essential tool.

The role of first-line leaders during joint field work

The real purpose of doing joint field work today is so your medical representatives won't need you on sales calls in the future. As a first-line leader, you should keep it in mind that the medical representatives are the internal customers. They expect value added service from their leaders during joint field work. So the ideal way would be to map the profile and needs of medical representatives and accordingly offer value added service to them. Below are some of your main roles during joint field work:

Catch medical representative doing right thing – The most important is to *catch your medical representative doing the right thing and praise.* This has been the best motivating factor of a medical representative. *'Acknowledge a job well done,'* medical representatives want to be told when they have done a good job. Use praise liberally and often.

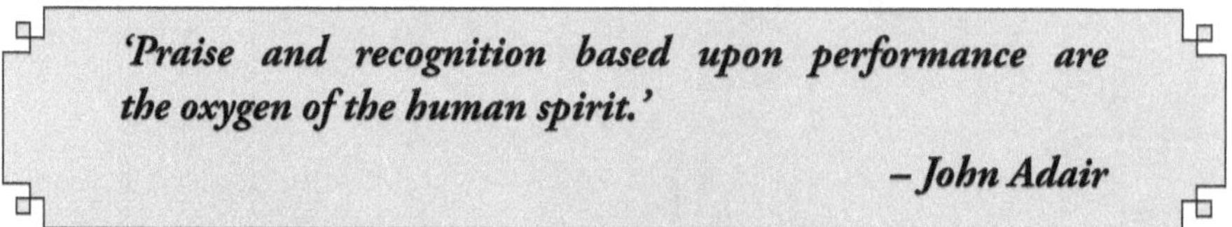

'Praise and recognition based upon performance are the oxygen of the human spirit.'

– John Adair

Discussion on correspondence – You should spend 10–15 minutes to discuss each correspondence with your medical representatives. There are several ways of correspondence like official email communication, newsletters, social media engagements and many more. If required, make them reply to those communications immediately.

Training on product knowledge – First observe the understanding levels of product knowledge and the way they explain the benefits and usage to healthcare professionals. Next is to take up products (one at a time) and give straight forward questions and reply with respect to composition, mode of action and how to convert doctors to your brand. In addition, you initiate and start discussing about the product with the doctors so that medical representatives can learn from the conversations and can make necessary changes in their next calls.

Develop communication of medical representatives – Communication is an important tool for medical representatives to create prescription demand. Communication is done through detailing of products to the doctors with clarity, pause, voice modulation, and punch. During detailing, it is also imperative to effectively communicate the benefits of our brands to doctors. You have to ensure that each medical representative is thorough with the detailing for every product under promotion. Do not take any medical representative for joint field work without ensuring that they are thorough with detailing of all products. In case, they are weak in detailing, then you should demonstrate the detailing and if required detail at certain doctor chambers and help them through such modelling activities. Effective communication is developed only through practice, and more practice.

Monitoring the implementation – Joint Field work is the platform to monitor the implementation. You can observe the detailing, sampling, input utilization and adherence to the brand matrix. Whenever needed, you can demonstrate how to implement the strategy designed by HO. For example; how to effectively communicate with the doctor and highlight a particular point.

Avoid supervisory bossy behavior like policing, constantly correcting which will lead to bitterness. You have to make your JFW constructive and fun. Do not be a pillion rider.

KEY POINTS: Joint Field Work

Time allocation: *Joint field work is a continuous process and you need to carry out the JFW every month. The number of joint field work days may vary based on the priorities. The allocation of number of days has to be planned in following three categories:*

- *Newly joined medical representative*
- *Weak territories*
- *Highly contributing territories*

Check list: *Before going to a territory you have to check the following and prepare your action plans.*

- *Monthly stocks and sales statements*
- *Field efforts of medical representative*
- *Sales figures, brand wise and month wise*
- *Campaign feedback*

Communication: *A clear communication has to be sent in advance to the medical representative, mentioning the number of days, places of JFW and objectives for your visit. If required, remind them on phone. The effectiveness of joint field work will depend upon the clarity of communication.*

Don't substitute the job of medical representative: *Often it happens that the first-line leader tries to compensate the lacunae of medical representatives by stepping into their shoes during the call to convert the doctors. The probable objective is to gain immediate prescriptions (short term goal) from the doctor rather than developing the medical representatives which is the actual long term goal.*

Work at least three days: *Whenever you are working with Medical representatives, work a minimum of three days at a stretch.*

- ***1st Day of JFW:*** *Discuss the objective of your present visit and make sure the work plan matches your objectives. Appreciate the good things that the medical representative has done on on-going assignments. Mostly observe and avoid unwanted interventions.*
- ***2nd Day of JFW:*** *Based on the observation made on the 1st day, discuss the areas of improvement and if required, you can demonstrate how things could be done. Again observe medical representative closely, if still needs improvement, ask to practice.*
- ***3rd Day of JFW:*** *On 3rd day, revisit the point discussed on 2nd day and let medical representative analyse the extent of success and failure. Encourage so that he/she will feel committed to the assignments.*

Advantages of joint field work

Joint field work conducted every month has many advantages. In fact, if JFW is carried out in professional manner, it will benefit medical representatives, first-line leaders as well as the organisation.

Benefit to the medical representatives

- Medical representatives get support to build their skills.
- They get a chance to show-off their skills.
- It is an opportunity for them to learn from their leaders.
- They also get support in generating more prescriptions.

Benefit to the first-line leaders

- Joint field work is an opportunity to establish your leadership.
- You can assess the happenings of market place.
- This is also an opportunity to praise your medical representatives.
- During JFW, you can build rapport with key customers.
- You can monitor the level of strategy implementation.

Benefit to the organisation

- Joint field work develops medical representatives, which is helping the organisation in getting better talent.
- First-line leader increases commitment of medical representatives towards the organisation.
- Joint field work reduces the attrition.
- Most importantly, joint field work ensures better productivity.

Three steps of joint field work

1. **Pre-call planning (Before the call)**

   Each success starts with planning. Pre-call planning is the foundation of the sales call. During joint field work, before entering doctor's chamber you clarify the followings:

- Doctor's information and prescribing habits.
- What was the response of the doctor in the last call?
- Whether the doctor is in any campaign?
- What are the inputs invested in recent past?
- Current support of the doctor from detailed RCPA.

Based on the above information, you plan the call based on the following questions:

- What is the objective of the call?
- What points do you want to make?
- What questions do you want to ask the doctor?
- What questions the doctor may ask and how to handle those questions?
- How to take commitment from the doctor?

Most importantly, both you and your medical representative mutually agree what role the medical representative will play and what role you will play.

2. **Observation (During the call)**

   There are two components:

   - **Observe the medical representative** – You have to observe the medical representative during the call. You should also check the level of implementation. Avoid unplanned intervention and let the medical representative be the hero of the call.
   - **Observe the doctor** – Doctors may not express their opinion about your brands or organisation but you can get a sense of it from their body language. Knowledge about body language (nor verbal communication) will help you to understand the signals conveyed by the doctor during the call.

3. **Post call analysis (After the call)**

   Post call analysis is the process of assessing and recording the result of the call, in order to plan the future calls. It is very essential to keep a record, because it is very difficult to remember what happened in each call.

After finishing every call, you set an objective for next call based on the following points:

- Whether the main points conveyed to the doctor?
- What was the response of the doctor?
- Whether is the closing done in a proper way?

After the call, you must praise your medical representative for doing the good things during the call. You should encourage your medical representative to analyse the call, let him/her come out with his/her ideas and then give your suggestions for improvement.

Control Measures

Controlling is one of the most important functions of a first-line leader to keep medical representatives on track. There are different stages of control measures. For example:

During joint field work

- Ask the retailer about the non-moving product and personally check the manufacturing date. This gives an idea on the prescription flow. The prescription flow is an indicator of a medical representative's work.
- Observe the way medical representative greets the chemist.
- You can observe the greeting and expressions of doctors during the representative's visit and also the behaviour of the receptionist.
- Sudden change in the tour programme and work in another territory can sometimes give you some indications.

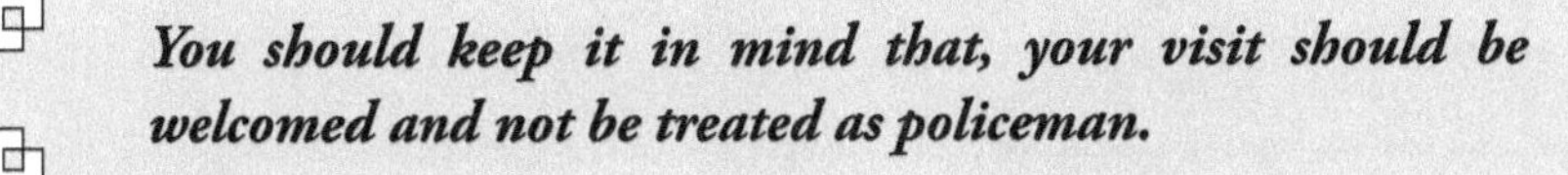

You should keep it in mind that, your visit should be welcomed and not be treated as policeman.

After joint field work

'Leadership is about making others better as a result of your presence and making sure that the impact lasts in your absence.' Leaving a lasting impression is a sign of effective leaders.

What's important as a leader is not what happens when you are there; it's what happens when you're not there. An effective leader is one who makes his/her presence felt even when he/she is absent. You cannot work for an entire month with one medical representative and it is very important for you to know what is happening in the territory. You can use the following reports:

Daily activity reports: The daily activity reports help you to analyse the activities of your medical representatives such as missed calls, missed doctors, visit frequencies, coverage and much more. Based on these reports, you can give feedback and suggestions for improvement on a regular basis.

Stock and sales statements: The stockist's stock and sales statements help you to analyse the secondary trend, new products movement and the inventory status.

Campaign feedback: Feedback on campaigns enables you to understand the current happenings in the territory. For example, input distribution status reflects the implementation of the strategies.

KEY POINTS: Control Measures

1. *Validate the brand matrix during JFW.*
2. *Monitor coverage as well as visit frequency. Communicate to your team on a weekly basis about missed doctors as well as missed calls.*
3. *It is a must for you to check the right communication of visual aid.*
4. *In case for those where the input utilization feedback is not satisfactory, you have to plan to distribute maximum inputs during JFW.*
5. *You must check thoroughly the expense statements of your medical representatives.*

Feedback from first-line leader to medical representative

> *'Feedback is the breakfast for champions.'*
>
> *– Kenneth Blanchard*

As a first-line leader, you need to give feedback to your medical representatives. Giving feedback is one of the hardest things for leaders. Humans are so emotional, and when their livelihood is at stake, they can be so sensitive to any feedback that comes from leaders. In our context, a feedback is the information sent to medical representatives based on their past role, so that they can adjust their current and future roles to achieve the desired results. Feedback should be given in such a way that the medical representatives truly benefit from it and the relationship between you and medical representatives become better. While you prepare feedback to be given to a medical representative, you must keep it in mind the following points:

Avoid judgements: Avoid judgemental statements such as 'Your performance is not good' or 'you don't know how to detail.' Rather you should discuss the symptoms and observation and let the medical representatives know that you are here to discuss what you feel.

Use examples: While giving feedback, drive the conversation using examples and mention what you would have done in that situation. Real life examples give more confidence and room for discussion.

Focus on the strength of medical representatives: Each medical representative has a set of strengths and weaknesses. While giving feedback, stay focused on the strengths, for example; share your observations about the things that the medical representative is doing really well.

Feedback is the stepping stones to success. There are three types of feedbacks:

Positive feedback: It consists of simple praise, but is even more powerful when you highlight why or how the medical representative did the good job. For example, "I appreciate your effort in making the new brand available in Apollo Hospital, which will serve the indoor patients and it will contribute to your secondary sale. Congrats."

Constructive feedback: Constructive feedback highlights how the medical representative could do better next time. It consists of areas of improvement with appropriate action plans. It is very essential to provide your medical representative with both types (Positive and Constructive) of feedback in order to improve and maintain quality performance.

Negative feedback: This is an inevitable part of being a leader, but something that needs to be treated very delicately. Leaders should be aware of this because one piece of negative feedback can overshadow the other positive feedback they give. Negative feedback is used to point out what the medical representatives did not do or how they fell short of the expected behaviours. Negative feedback can create demotivation to the medical representatives. You should convey negative feedback in a positive manner (with empathetic concern) without demotivating the medical representative. For example:

> *Last year your call average was 10. But since the last two months, it has come down to 8. If you are facing any difficulty, then feel free to share with me, so that I can help you to overcome it in future.*

> ***'Researchers found that leaders who gave negative feedback with empathetic concern got better responses from their employees.'***

Medical representatives respond more positively to criticism and are more likely to take feedback to heart when they feel their leader cares about their well-being and wants them to improve. Followings are some of tips of giving negative feedback:

1. Always condemn actions, not medical representatives. Make sure the medical representative understands that any criticism is about the work and not the individual.
2. Your body language and tone of voice affect how the feedback is perceived. Even if you as a leader can handle negative feedback, you should assume that the team member is incredibly sensitive and will be affected by the feedback.
3. Always start and end with a positive note. Suppose you schedule a 30-minute meeting, start by highlighting a few good things that the medical representative has done recently, and end by reminding what a valuable he or she is.
4. Schedule a meeting so that they can mentally prepare themselves for the feedback, they'll be able to handle it much better.
5. Whenever they need help for improvement, you should be ready with very specific recommendations (with examples) on what they can do.

CASE STUDY

Mr. Rahul aged 23, working as a medical representative in a same territory since joining. Rahul has 200 doctors in his list and 50 of whom are VVIP doctors. You have rated Rahul as a satisfactory sales performer. Rahul understands company plan and territory goals. He has a very good relationship with most of the KOLs. He needs supervision and help in planning. You believe that Rahul has the capability to improve his productivity.

You have three days JFW with him from Monday and arrange to meet him at your hotel at his HQ town for breakfast on Monday at 8.00 am. On your last JFW, the conclusion you reached was his performance was acceptable but not up to the potential. Rahul needed help.

Circumstances 1: *Rahul arrives at 8.30 am; apologetically explaining and at the same time informing you that he has an appointment with the purchase officer of the New Town Hospital at 9 am. Normally, in the first one hour of your visit you review planned activities for next three days of JFW and at the same time receive feedback on the progress on your assignments if any. What course of action do you take?*

1. *Tell Rahul to change the appointment with the purchase officer and continue the review.*
2. *Give Rahul a talk on the time management.*
3. *Meet the purchase officer at 9 am.*

Circumstances 2: *On your way to hospital, you ask Rahul about the objective of the call. He informs you that it is his call for new product availability at New Town Hospital. You recall from your previous JFW that New Town Hospital hasn't yet cracked for a new product. You also recall that Rahul is trying to make his new product available in this hospital. What do you do?*

1. *Ask him about his progress in New Town Hospital.*
2. *Since you have not met the purchase officer, ask Rahul about him.*
3. *Say nothing.*

Circumstances 3: *Your joint call with the purchase officer concludes at 9.30 am. Rahul's next appointment is at 11am. You ask Rahul if this is a suitable time to the earlier review session. Rahul agrees. In addition to the review, you also need to discuss the call with the purchasing officer. What do you do?*

1. *Use some valuable time to discuss the call on purchasing officer.*
2. *Wait until end of day's work.*
3. *Wait until the end of your visit (Till Wednesday evening) and discuss the call during the whole field work review session.*

Circumstances 4: *During review, Rahul tells you about his difficulty of making new products available in few more private hospitals. As you listen to him, it becomes obvious to you that Rahul needs and wants help in this area. Which strategy should you employ?*

1. *Offer your opinion as to what would be the best course of action best on the situation.*
2. *Provide Rahul with specific information that he lacks or has not used.*
3. *Give Rahul specific information and show him how to use that information.*
4. *Help him explore the problems and alternative ways of dealing with them so that he can decide what to do with them.*

Work Relationship

> ***High performance medical representatives are dependent on high quality relationship with their first-line leaders.***

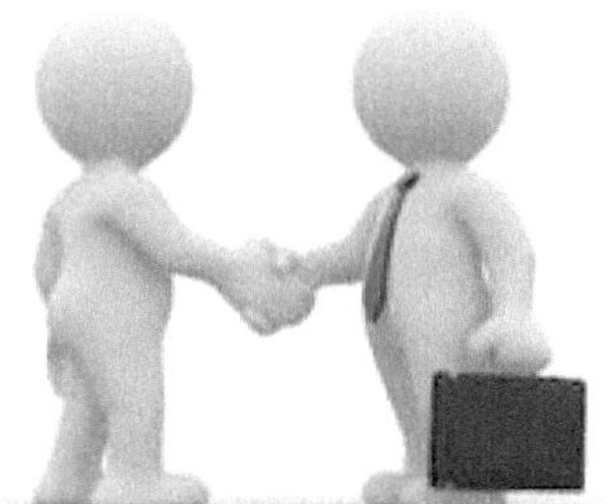

'The deeper your relationship, the stronger your leadership.' Successful business is built upon a strong work relationship, which means the stronger the bond between you and your medical representatives, the stronger the result. You will enjoy your work if you have a good relationship with your medical representatives. Below are some of the ways by which you can improve your work relationship –

Develop a positive attitude – Your attitude towards joint field work is very important to build a very good work relationship. Avoid negative thoughts and criticism. Be less judgemental and more accepting of your medical representatives.

Avoid jumping to the conclusion – Jumping to conclusion is something we are all very good at. We see something and we make an assumption. We may be right or we may be wrong. Jumping to conclusions to a situation without knowing the whole story can cause misunderstanding. Do not provide quick, easy solutions to complicated situations. Even if the issue looks so simple, you need to take the time to listen, and then think of the best response.

Improve your communication – No relationship can survive without healthy communication. Effective communications can help you build strong working relationships with your medical representatives. Listen carefully and completely; when medical representative finished, state your understanding to ensure there is no misinterpretation. Communicate with respect in every interaction regardless of whether you like the person.

Resolves conflict early – Conflict is a part of a relationship and arises from the differences. If it is not resolved early it can harm relationships. By resolving conflict early and positively, you can keep your personal and professional relationship strong and growing. Resolving a conflict is a skill which you need to develop. Your ability to keep calm and focused is essential for resolving a conflict. Always be in control of your emotions so that you can effectively communicate your needs without threatening, frightening your medical representative.

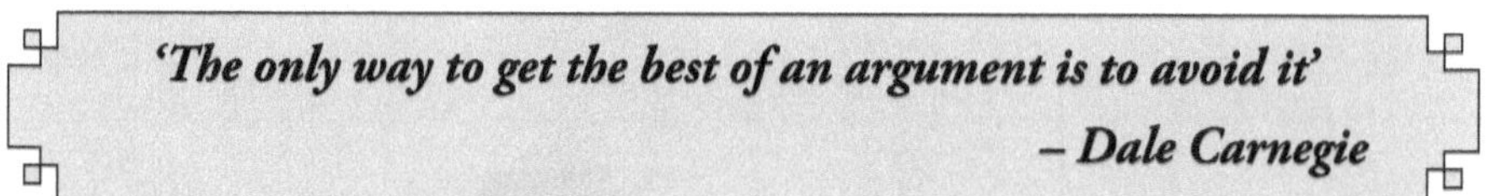

'The only way to get the best of an argument is to avoid it'

– Dale Carnegie

Set boundaries – Developing friendship is a natural process. However, it is important to set boundaries to ensure that friendship does not interfere with the work. Some medical representatives will be tempted to take advantage of your relationship if you're too friendly with them. You do need to get the balance right between being a friend and being the superior.

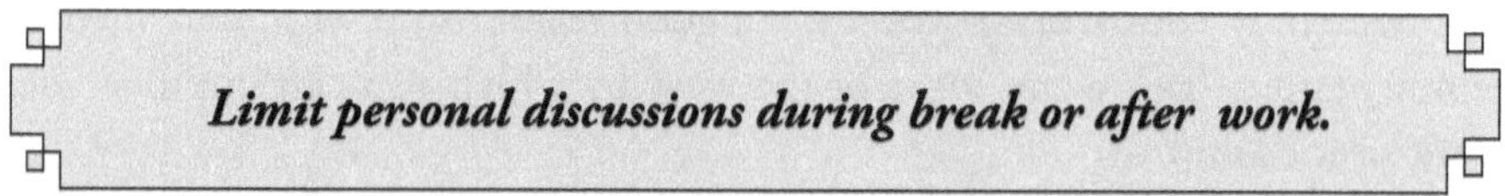

Limit personal discussions during break or after work.

Accept personal and cultural difference – People come to work in an organisation from different cultural and social backgrounds. Cultural difference is the significant uniqueness of each member in a team. Every culture has different values and worldviews, which can make it challenging for leaders to work together. You must be aware of diversity, and how to manage it to the best effect. When you accept this diversity, you acknowledge and welcome him or her into your environment, regardless of whether you share his/her cultural values, characteristics or experiences.

- *Be accepting; always look at the things from other's perspective.*
- *Encourage your medical representatives to take an interest in one another's belief.*
- *Leaders, who welcome this diversity, are successful.*

Induction of a new medical representative

A newly joined medical representative is a vital asset to the organisation. He/she is like a new born baby who needs special care and attention. Developing and grooming of the newly joined medical representative is one of the most important responsibilities of a first-line leader. Induction is a structured and supportive method of introducing newly recruited medical representatives to their new roles and working environments. It should familiarise about the culture, accepted practices and performance standards of the organisation. Induction provides a great opportunity to stimulate engagement in medical representatives.

Usually, field induction has to be planned immediately after the new medical representative completes his/her basic classroom training from head office. Organising and delivering a thorough field induction programme is an important activity for you as a first-line leader. The objective of a field induction is to achieve maximum working efficiency in the shortest possible time. During this period, you work for the first time with the medical representative; this is the chance to make your first impression. Your first impressions last the importance of good field induction. Effective field induction has a measurable return on investment; not only through decreased turnover costs but by increasing productivity of the medical representative. Before giving the field induction you have to ensure that the new medical representative receives the followings:

1. Detailing bag
2. Visual aid and detailing guide
3. Doctor list, chemist list
4. Promotional materials, like samples, LBLs
5. Strategy guide
6. Incentive circulars
7. Holiday list
8. Standard tour plan and standard fare chart
9. Target and achievement sheets
10. Stationery (All the reporting formats)

Field induction of a newly joined medical representative is not a one-day event; for an effective field induction, you should work with him for a minimum of six days. Here are the guidelines to be followed on each day of the field induction.

DAY 1 – The first day of field work is very important. Welcome and greet the medical representative so that he/she feels comfortable. You should spend a couple of hours with him before starting the field work. This time is to be utilised for explaining him the followings:

- Major towns and ex and out stations of the territory.
- Doctor list including VVIP and important doctors.
- Strategies and on-going campaign if any.
- Important hospitals and top chemists.
- Importance of daily call reporting.

You have to check the detailing before you proceed to the field.

The first day field work must start with RCPA. The actual work should be taken up by you. The newly joined medical representative would be asked to observe, encouraged to seek clarification and follow the same. This will build his confidence. You need to demonstrate how to set objectives for the call from the RCPA. You must explain the brand matrix. You should open the order book at every chemist and demonstrate personal order booking. You must make a note of all the information of RCPA in the dairy or note book. Also make note of doctor visited, product detailed, input given etc.

At the end of first day's field work, you help him to submit the DCR. This must be done after each day's field work. Every day you should give him some assignments based on his skills and knowledge.

DAY 2 – Welcome and ask about first day's experience. Discuss features and benefits of all the brands as well as how to handle objections. Evaluate the product knowledge as well as knowledge of competitor brands. The second day induction involves the followings:

- Listen to the detailing of newly joined medical representative.
- Ask question about compositions, competitors.
- Brief him the work plan for the day.
- You and newly joined medical representative should do alternate chemist and doctor calls.
- Catch him doing the right thing.

DAY 3 – Discuss objection handling techniques and how to close a call successfully. Explain the importance of closing a call and discuss different closing techniques. Discuss about the importance of pre-call planning and post call analysis. Demonstrate how to set the objective of a call based on RCPA. Immediately after each call, analyse the call. Motivate by highlighting the good things done by the medical representative during the call. On third day, the first call should be done by you and the later calls should be done by newly joined medical representatives.

DAY 4 – Explain about monthly tour plan, standard tour plan. Show him how to prepare day's plans as well as master customer coverage plans. Discuss about strategy implementation and its importance. All calls should be done by the medical representative. Catch him doing the right thing and praise.

DAY 5 – Share with him the product wise primary and secondary sales of the HQ and provide the stock and sales statements. Show him how to prepare secondary compilation. Discuss targets sheet and contribution of each brand. Discuss how to achieve brand wise objective by dividing into number of doctors, number of prescriptions etc. Also explain the followings:

Secondary sales – importance of Rx generation.

Primary sales – importance of secondary sales.

Closing stocks – implication of high inventory stocks, transit stocks.

DAY 6 – Summarise the whole work in terms of product knowledge, detailing, strategy implantation, RCPA as well as timely submission of daily reports. Appraise and offer your suggestions for improvement. Leave him with a sense of direction and high degree of motivation. Before leaving the territory, discuss on areas of improvements and never make any negative comment.

Effective field induction ensures that newly joined medical representatives become integrated both functionally and socially into the organisation and its environment. Communicate frequently to encourage and to give the medical representative a feeling of security.

> ***'We focus first on the people and how we incorporate them into our company, and then we focus on how to drive the business.'***
>
> ***– John Chambers***

CHAPTER 4

MOTIVATION

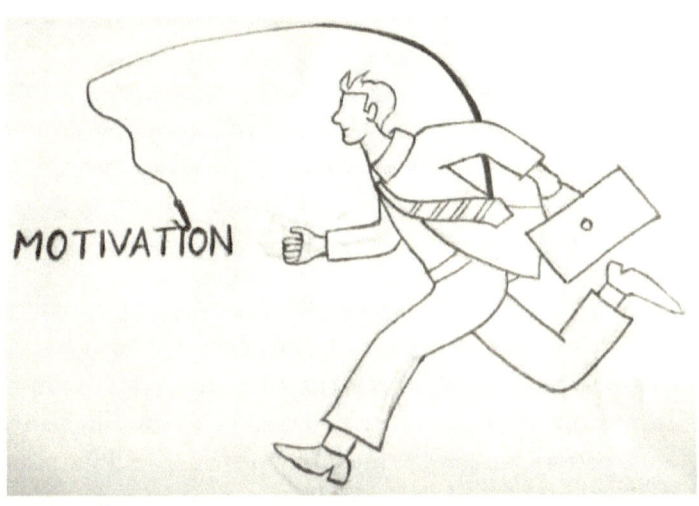

> ***'If communication is sister to leadership, then Motivation is brother.'***
>
> ***– John Adair***

Motivation is the word derived from the word *'motive' which* derives from the Latin verbs *'movere,'* to move. So a motive is something that moves you in action. Motivation is a complex and least understood subject; because it is an internal feeling, cannot be observed directly. It is the most effective instrument for getting things done from human beings. Human beings don't change their state of affairs until a force is applied on them. This force is motivation, the force that causes people to act or behave in an unexpected way.

There are two types of motivation; intrinsic (we want to) and extrinsic (we have to). Intrinsic motivators include recognition, social status, confidence and self-actualisation needs which are related to inner aspects of a person. You can feel motivated internally only when you have burning desires to achieve. Extrinsic motivation is external in nature. Extrinsic motivation comes through supervisors, companions, parents or spouse. For an extrinsic motivated person, work is only a means that needs to be done in order to get the rewards associated with the job.

Motivation is the most important function of management to create willingness among the employees to perform in the best of their abilities. It's a condition that stimulates desire to work and do a good job at it. Motivated employees give their best to the organisation. They stay loyal and committed to the organisation.

> ***'Leadership is the ability of a single individual through his or her actions to motivate others to high levels of achievement.'***
>
> ***– F. G. Buck Rodgers***

In order to attain goals and achieve success in any organisation, leaders must know how to motivate their team members. Leadership includes the ability to motivate and inspire others. For a first-line leader motivation is a process of stimulating medical representatives into action. Motivation plays a vital role in the performance of the medical representative. It inspires medical representatives to stay focused on their job and work towards achieving their goals. Motivation seems to be a simple function of management in books; but in reality, it is more challenging because of the followings:

Nobody can motivate anybody: Motivation is really the spirit of a person. It is like the fuel in the car that starts the engine. A person gets motivated or demotivated solely because of himself. Practically *'you can't motivate people, you can only create a context in which people are motivated.'*

> ***'Leaders create a work environment in which people feel terrific about themselves'***

Motivation is a continuous process: To motivate a person is easy but to keep the person motivated is not easy. Motivation is continuous process rather than a one shot affair; because an individual has unlimited wants and needs. For example, in our context, it has been observed that in a cycle meeting, medical representatives get motivated to do whatever is asked for. However as soon as they reach their territories, the enthusiasm evaporates. *'It is like blowing a balloon, if we do not tie a knot, the air will go out.'* Hence motivation is not a one-time booster. Motivation is like fire, unless we keep adding fuel it dies out. Motivation is what keeps the fire burning.

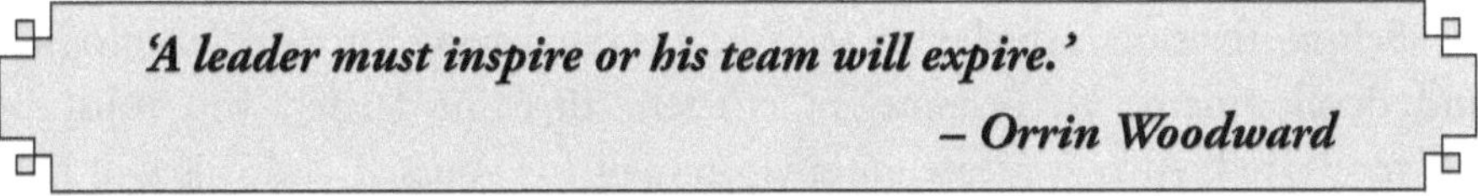

'A leader must inspire or his team will expire.'

– Orrin Woodward

Both required 'Money and Job Satisfaction': Everyone wants money, no doubt. Money rewards are found very effective to motivate medical representatives. This can be in the form of incentives, promotions, increments in the salaries, special allowances, performance based bonus etc. Money is better at attracting and retaining people than at influencing their behaviour. Money is not only reason that makes people perform extraordinary tasks. Fortunately, there are factors that motivate people more than money; for example, Job satisfaction is so important and the absence of it leads to lethargy and reduced organisational commitment. Job satisfaction is an emotional response to a job situation. As such it cannot be seen, it can only be inferred. In fact, *'money and job satisfactions are the two wings of a bird; one is enough for survival but to fly high both are required.'*

Four Rules of Motivation

'An Employee's motivation is a direct result of the sum of interaction with his or her manager.'

– Bob Nelson

Motivation plays an important role in productivity, quality, and speed of work. When employees lack motivation, these factors are greatly affected. Followings are the four rules of motivation:

1. Be motivated yourself

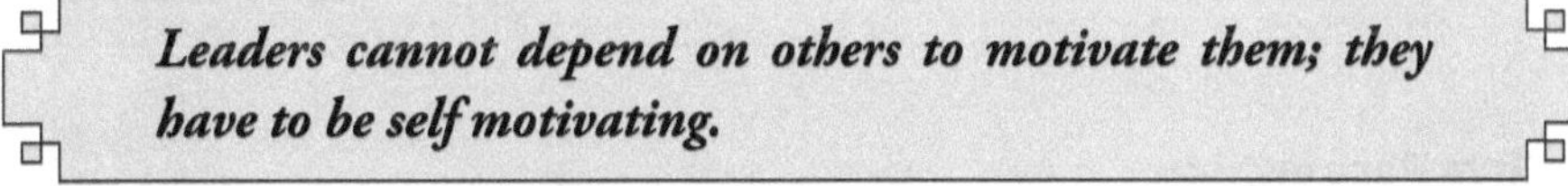

Leaders cannot depend on others to motivate them; they have to be self motivating.

Only a motivated leader can motivate others. The golden rule of motivation is that if you are self- motivated, only then you can motivate others to achieve their goals and to harmonise their personal goals with the common goals of the organisation.

Self-motivation is the key to success. It is the driving force behind progress and development. To become an efficient first-line leader, you must be self-motivated. Always create an environment for yourself and this will help you to become more motivated to achieve your dreams and goals.

- *Think of your accomplishments and you fill your mind with elevating and inspiring information, it will keep you motivated.*
- *Your commitment is very important in motivating your team. Commitment moves through tough decisions into action. In fact, real commitments commence to transform you.*
- *'Motivation is a virus; it is caught, not taught.'*

2. Be a role model

> ***'Be the change that you want to see in the world.'***
>
> ***– Mahatma Gandhi***

A role model is someone who serves as an example, whose behaviour is emulated by other people and consistently leads by example. Being a role model is a powerful management tool. Being a role model is the key motivator that influences people in reaching their goals. You should set a good example to ensure medical representatives grow and achieve their goals effectively. *'People do what people see'*; medical representatives watch closely the action, habit, behaviour and character of their leaders and then try to imbibe in their styles. It does not matter what you communicate, but your action which actually motivates your team.

> ***'The best example of leadership is leadership by example.'***
>
> ***– Jerry McClain***

3. Give Recognition

> ***'Recognition is the most inexpensive motivational technique available to management.'***

'Appreciation is a fundamental human need.' Everyone values positive recognition. The fact is *'what gets rewarded gets done'* and people respond to appreciation expressed through recognition of their good work because it confirms their work is valued. Medical representatives expect that their successes to be rewarded, praised and celebrated. The cost of recognition is quite small and the benefits are large when implemented effectively.

> ***'Appreciation can make a day. Even change a life. Your willingness to put it into words is all that is necessary.'***
>
> ***– Margaret Cousins***

4. Give Positive Feedback

> ***'One of the most tried-and-true forms of management is feedback.'***
>
> ***– Dr. Christopher Lee***

Feedback is essential for chasing goals. Feedback includes advice, praise, evaluation and criticism as well. In an organisation, one of the best ways to help employees perform better is to give them feedback. Medical representatives need regular feedback to know how they are doing and to keep on track. Positive feedback can generate wins for the first-line leaders. Highlighting the strengths of a medical representative can help generate a sense of accomplishment and motivation. To make your feedback even more powerful and productive it is essential to understand the emotions of the medical representatives, how they may be feeling. Make sure to focus on the future; what can your medical representatives do to move forward?

Not giving feedback on progress to medical representatives leads to demotivation. Always keep them informed because they want to know what's really going on.

Maslow's Needs: The Theory of Human Motivation

Maslow's theory of motivation is called the "hierarchy of needs." This theory is a classical illustration of human motivation. Abraham Maslow stated that people are motivated to achieve certain needs. This theory is based on the assumption that there is a hierarchy of five needs within each individual. When one need is fulfilled a person seeks to fulfil the next one, and so on. According to Maslow every human being has five basic needs.

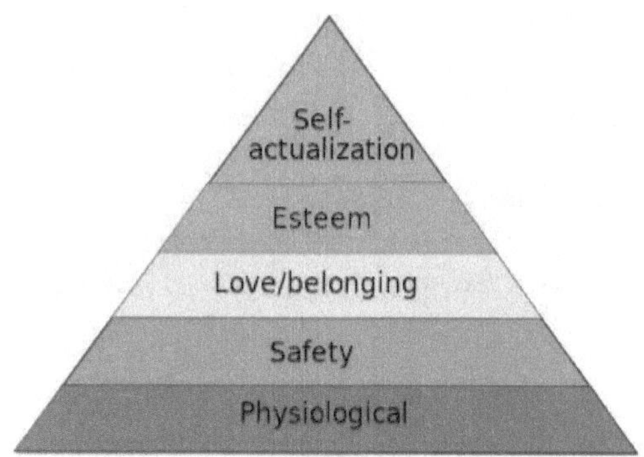

Fig: Maslow's hierarchy of needs

1. **Physiological needs** – Physiological needs are the physical requirements for human survival. These are the basic needs of air, water, food, clothing and shelter. In other words, physiological needs are the needs for basic amenities of life. If a person becomes chronically short of food and water he or she becomes dominated by the desire to eat and drink, and concern for other needs tends to be swept away. Physiological needs are the most important; they should be met first.
2. **Safety needs** – Once the physiological needs get fulfilled, a new set of needs i.e. safety needs take precedence. Safety needs include physical, environmental and emotional safety and protection. For instance – job security, financial security, protection from animals, family security, health security, etc.
3. **Social needs** – After physiological and safety needs are fulfilled, the third level of human needs is interpersonal and involves feelings of belongingness such as friend, family etc. Humans need to love and be loved by others. These needs are intrinsic to our human nature.

4. **Esteem needs** – Esteem needs are the typical human desire to be accepted and valued by others. Most people have a need for stable self-respect and self-esteem. Esteem needs are of two types: internal esteem needs (self-respect, confidence, competence, achievement and freedom) and external esteem needs (recognition, power, status, attention and admiration).

5. **Self-actualization needs** – Unlike lower level needs, this need never fully satisfied. Only a few can reach this level. This includes the urge to become what you are capable of becoming/what you have the potential to become. It includes the need for growth and self-contentment. It also includes a desire for gaining more knowledge, social – service, creativity and being aesthetic. What a man can be, he must be. Example – a musician must make music, a poet must write.

Maslow classified these needs into higher and lower levels.

1. **Lower levels:** The physiological and the safety needs constituted the lower levels and these are satisfied externally.

2. **Higher levels:** The social, esteem, and self-actualisation needs constituted the higher levels. These higher level needs are generally satisfied internally, i.e., within an individual.

According to Maslow, once the lower levels of need are substantially satisfied, an individual moves up the hierarchy and the next levels of need predominate. If you want to motivate someone, you need to understand where exactly the person currently is on the hierarchy and focus on satisfying the needs at or above the particular level. Understanding people's motives, their reasons for doing something is the key to becoming a good leader.

Maslow's theory has an inherent appeal and obvious relevance for first-line leaders. Each medical representative has basic needs that must be met before they can perform at their best. You need to ensure that these needs are satisfied and the medical representatives are both psychologically and emotionally free.

The challenge before first-line leaders is to determine at which position the medical representative is in Maslow's hierarchy of needs. There are medical representatives who come to work to earn money and have no desire either to get on with others, or earn promotion. Some medical representatives have a personal challenge and sense of achievement. Few of them work to gain experience to get a promotion. For others it may be a combination of these. Place them on Maslow's pyramid to identify their actual motivational needs. Maslow's theory is very popular, particularly among practising leaders because it is based on an intuitive logic and is easy to understand and relate to.

KEY POINTS: Important Motivators

'True motivation comes from achievement, personal development, job satisfaction, and recognition' - Frederick Herzberg

Achievements - *Sense of achievement lasts long and the sense of achievement itself motivates a person.*

Your job is not to motivate medical representatives to get them to achieve; instead, you should provide opportunities for them to achieve, so that they will become motivated.

Personal Growth - *'Employees will always perform at their best when the environment is conducive to growth.'*

If your medical representatives find their job as a source of growth in their skills, they will feel motivated. You should help your medical representatives to develop their skills, which will ultimately lead them to achieve their respective goals.

Recognition and Appreciation - *'One of the deepest drives of human nature is the desire to be appreciated.'*

Study reveals that '79% of employees quit their jobs due to lack of appreciation.' When medical representatives receive validation and sincere appreciation, they are energised to do their best.

How to motivate medical representative

> ***'In motivating people, you have to engage their minds and their hearts.'***
>
> ***– Rupert Murdoch***

One of the easiest ways to motivate people is to *'catch them doing something right and recognise them for it.'* Many medical representatives do not know exactly what motivates them in the field. There are instances where many potential medical representatives left the organisation due to lack of motivation. Knowing different needs of medical representative is very essential. You must have a thorough knowledge of motivational factors for your medical representatives.

To motivate medical representatives to peak performance, continually make them feel important and valuable.

You must learn how to motivate medical representatives. You must be aware of their needs and wants. These needs and wants are different with different medical representatives and are different in different stages of their career. Following are a few ways to motivate a medical representative:

Specific approach: The fact is that your medical representatives are all unique and are therefore motivated by different things. One rule doesn't apply to all; moreover, every individual has a different personality. You have to learn the personalities of each of your medical representative and adjust your approach accordingly. You need to ask questions to learn where their motivation stems from. You should provide all necessary resources and training needed by them to do the job. By doing so, they will perceive that you care for their well-being and they will feel motivated and will work better.

Often leaders commit mistakes in handling all medical representatives in the same manner. What motivates one does not necessarily motivate the other. You need different strokes for different folks.

Avoid favouritism: Motivation is an emotional issue, not a rational one, and you can't tell your medical representatives to get excited about work if they don't feel it. While assessing medical representatives, don't be biased as it may frustrate the purpose. Favouritism and bias are counterproductive in motivating a medical representative. The focus should be on performance.

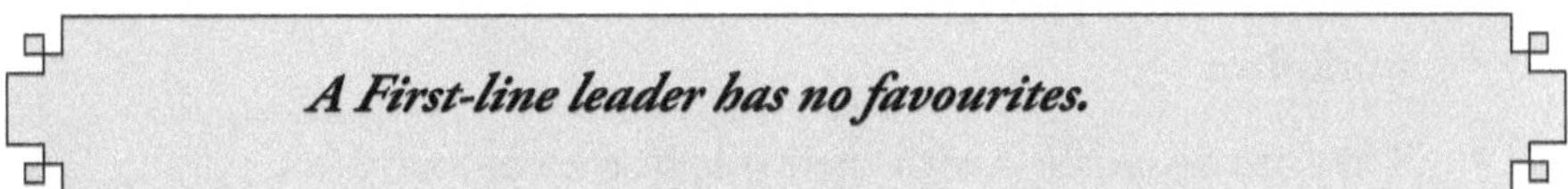
A First-line leader has no favourites.

Active listening: The greatest motivational act that a first-line leader can do for medical representatives is listening to them. When they come to you and share their problems, immediately stop everything and listen to them, there is nothing more important than that. You use techniques of active listening so that the medical representatives feel motivated.

Lead from the front: Leading from the front is where the leader sets the pace, destination and direction. '*Leadership is like moving a string. You cannot move it by pushing from behind; what you have to do is get ahead and pull.*' Leading from the front is leading by example; and it is the most powerful tool for positively influencing change in other people.

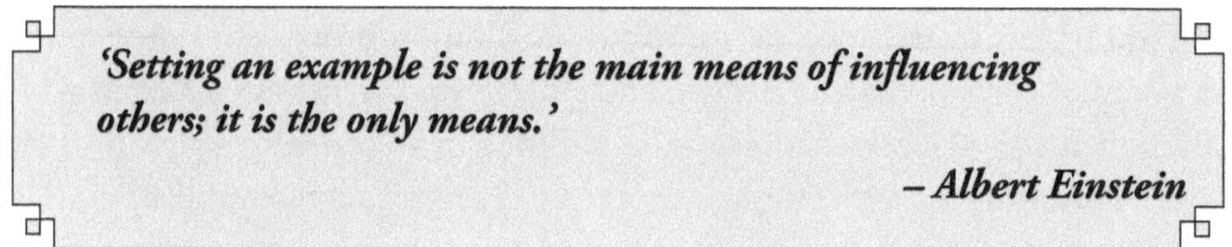

'Setting an example is not the main means of influencing others; it is the only means.'

– Albert Einstein

Medical representatives look to you for direction and guidance and they expect you to set an example for them to follow in their footsteps. Talk to them on a regular basis. Are they clear on the objectives? What are the challenges? How can you help, or what resources can you bring? Look for ways that your skills can compliment your medical representatives.

Who are demotivated medical representatives?

There are medical representatives who constantly need supervision because they don't have the initiative to work on their own. They rely on what their first-line leaders tell them before they make a move. They are demotivated medical representatives. They display following behaviours:

- They don't care about business goals or quality of the work they provide.
- When there's a problem, they complain, put the blame on others.
- They try to escape by passing the responsibility to others.
- They perform poorly and demonstrate negative behaviour in the workplace.
- They are dissatisfied with their role in the company.

Demotivated medical representatives carry a negative perception about everything that comes their way. They can be unproductive, adding to the costs of the organisation. It is very essential to recognise the sign of demotivation of the medical representatives. It is not an easy task to recognise because the symptoms of demotivation are not always a sad and depressed face. Recognising the warning signs of demotivation early and addressing them quickly, can encourage medical representatives in feeling comfort and also can reduce attrition.

KEY POINTS: Signs of demotivation

- *Medical representatives will spread negativity all around them.*
- *Productivity decreases gradually over a period of time.*
- *Not regular in the field.*
- *Leaving early and coming late to field is also a sign. They could invent a lie, just to stay away from work.*
- *Sometimes physically present but mentally not. They are preoccupied with other work and show interest in other work rather their own work.*
- *Some medical representatives always argue with their superior about trivial matters.*
- *They have no regard for their first-line leaders and flaunt the systems of the organisation without a fear of consequences.*
- *Negative body language of the medical representatives.*

There are many more signs, each relevant differently and in different extremities according to their contexts. A careful observation can be beneficial for the first-line leaders.

Reason for Demotivation

Demotivation is contagious; like *'one spoiled apple can spoil the whole basket.'* Even one demotivated medical representative can quickly succeed in demotivating others too. So, it's important for you to be aware of it, recognise and tackle it without delay. To tackle the demotivation effectively, you must know the cause of it. Following are some common causes of demotivation.

1. Poor leadership

Poor leadership can have several negative effects on the medical representatives. Poor leadership also leads to frustration in medical representatives which may be associated with poor performance, thus leading to demotivation. For example:

Lack of directions: Without a direction, medical representatives are aimless. It is essential for you to set the direction for your medical representatives so that they remain motivated. Medical representatives if not given direction periodically, they will be confused and dissatisfied, and this dissatisfaction can lead to demotivation.

Lack of recognition and rewards:

> ***'People work for money but go the extra mile for recognition, praise and rewards.'***
>
> ***– Dale Carnegie***

Recognition and rewards increases self-esteem and can create a feeling of accomplishment. Lack of recognition results in decline in productivity as well as increase the rate of attrition. You should always hunt for good behaviour. It is easy to catch someone doing wrong, but it needs a positive attitude to *'catch people doing things right.'* It is fact that the sooner a leader praises good behaviour, the more likely it is to be repeated.

> ***'Recognition delayed is recognition denied.'***

Micromanagement: This is a management style, where a first-line leader closely supervises or controls every work of medical representatives. It will be difficult to progress fast if you micromanage every little thing and not let your team grow and develop. The main reason for demotivation is that micromanagement discourages team members from taking decisions and resists delegating work. Medical representatives would feel stress instead of feeling empowered and they start performing poorly.

Lack of Empathy – Empathy is the ability to share other people's emotions. The better you feel what someone else is feeling, the more likely you can help them when they are in a difficult situation. As a leader when you put yourself in your team member's shoes, you start appreciating the hardship they face and will be in a position to provide them with the appropriate solution. Lack of empathy can lead to misunderstanding which ultimately leads to demotivation.

> ***'Never criticise a man till you have walked a mile in his shoes.'***

2. Poor sales achievements

Motivation is a huge part of sales achievements. Like athletes, medical representatives perform at their highest level only when fully motivated, incentivised and celebrated for their work. The level of motivation towards the job decides the achievements. If the achievements of medical representatives keep on being low quite a long time, they will certainly get demotivated. You have to find out the reason for poor sales achievements. There are many factors of poor performance which lead to the demotivation of the medical representative, for example:

- Medical representatives want interesting work environment where they are given responsibility, autonomy, challenges and the opportunity to learn. However inappropriate working conditions lead to dissatisfaction.
- In cases, when the territory targets are made without considering the realities, it affects the achievements which ultimately lead to the demotivation.
- The sales achievement of a medical representative depends on what their superior expects from them. Low expectation from first-line leader results in poor performance which leads to demotivation. Perhaps, no organisation can perform so well without the leader expecting a lot from the team members and pushing it to get the results.

> ***'High expectations lead to high results.'***

3. Conflict

Conflict can be described as friction or differences in opinions or incompatibilities. Conflicts become a part of our day to day business. At times conflict can be healthy, as long as it is discussed and a conclusion is reached. Clashing on personalities or opposing viewpoints can actually bring new ideas. How do you know when there is a conflict that must be addressed? Be alert!

> *Key Points: Signals of conflict*
>
> - *You find yourself reacting angrily to a suggestion. You discount the opinion of your team members.*
> - *You have stopped listening and are waiting for opportunity to jump in and disagree.*
> - *After trying to common ground, you cannot find a mutually acceptable solution.*
> - *You feel your priorities are more important.*

However, conflict in the workplace can be detrimental as it creates a lot of demotivation in the team members. When conflict arises, it can cause medical representatives to feel insecure about their place in and value to the organisation. They will feel that what is most important to them has been dishonoured. To resolve the conflict, you need to take steps and find an acceptable outcome. You should handle the conflict professionally and productively. The key to resolve conflict is not to run and hide. It's not to become combative. Rather, it is best dealt with by followings:

- *Accept the fact that conflict will occur. This will be the first step to resolve it.*
- *Conflict must be addressed immediately before it can grow bigger.*
- *Always seek to deal with issues, not with emotion.*
- *You need to focus more time on the issues related to productivity and meeting deadlines than on conflict resolution.*
- *Encourage the opinion of your medical representatives.*
- *Practice actively listening.*

- *Do not blame medical representatives, encourage ownership of the problems and solutions.*
- *Take a decision considering the facts and ensure medical representative is committed to work accordingly.*

Arguments cannot prove who is right or who is wrong; they just support self-images and create firmness in relationships. Hence it is better to discuss things transparently instead of arguing endlessly.

SITUATION

When a Medical Representative Seems Demotivated

Being human, at different points in our lives, we become demotivated for a while. Generally, this demotivation is temporary and we regain our enthusiasm for our work. What is not acceptable, however, is chronic demotivation that leads to poor sales achievements.

It's important for you to observe the medical representative's past behaviour before labelling them as demotivated. You have to identify the followings:

- *When the change in behaviour began?*
- *Was it gradual decline or there was a specific event that triggered it?*
- *Are there any recent conflicts?*
- *Have you changed your leadership style?*
- *Do you suspect any personal problems?*

The answers of the above will help you in handling the demotivation. When you find a medical representative getting demotivated and when you have your discussion; be very specific about what you have noticed and impact on the sales achievements. Your body language should convey the message that you care about their well-being and are not solely focused on the bottom line. Encourage them to open up and talk about what is not going well and why lack of motivation has set in.

- *If the cause of demotivation is work related, explore the ways to overcome the obstacles. Be creative and search for novel approaches to promote job function.*
- *If the cause lies in the personal issues, don't attempt to play non-professional psychologist yet at the same time offer possible help.*

There are no fixed rules to motivate a demotivated medical representative. It's actually your leadership skills which bring changes. *Following are some of the tips which can be helpful in handling a demotivated medical representative.*

- *Conduct a place where you discuss with him freely without any disturbance.*
- *Initiate the discussion with some broad remarks. Instead of referring to the issue yourself, let him/her reflect upon it.*
- *Depending upon the comments, ask the reason for the changes and instead of giving an answer, request him/her to suggest options.*
- *Once the medical representative acknowledges your viewpoint, spend some time reviewing clear goals and offering help so that he/she can feel that you care. It is important to make clear exactly what your performance related expectations are.*
- *Once both of you go to an accord for improving the behaviour, settle a suitable time period for behaviour modification.*
- *No one is great at every job; give them an opportunity to come with flying colours.*
- *Be empathetic and neutral.*

Chapter 5

COMMUNICATION SKILLS

'Communication is called the sister of leadership; effective leadership is to learn communication skills for working with others.'

Communication is an important part of our life. Communication is a transfer of thoughts, opinion or information from one person to another. The word communication has been derived from the Latin word *communis*, meaning 'common.' Communication is the art of being understood.

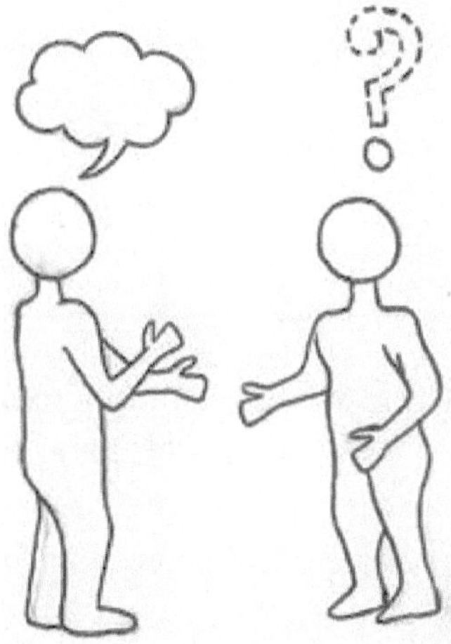

'Communication is not what we talk, but the response that we get. Communication requires response. The response ensures receipt of the message.'

Communication is not just the actual word you use; perhaps we can also communicate without words. Communication skills ensure that you have the ability to communicate both verbally and non-verbally. The moment we come into contact with some other person, we actually start communicating with that person. A total communication involves verbal words, tone and body language (non-verbal communication). The greater part of your message made up of non-verbal hints/signals, tone of voice and listening. An understanding of how communication works can help us to understand and improve.

According to Dr. Albert Mehrabian, 55% of our communication is non- verbal, 38% related to the tone and only 7% is verbal. You need to be flexible in all three elements of communication; words, tone and non-verbal.

Communication is the most important management tool. Leadership starts with good communication with people. First-line leaders motivate, encourage and inspire their medical representatives. They also train them, share new ideas and negotiate. These activities have one thing in common; they all require effective communication. Effective communication skills are an important aspect of any leader. ***Almost 85 percent success of a leader depends on how effectively he or she communicates.***

'Developing excellent communication skills is absolutely essential to effective leadership.'

– Gilbert Amelio

Communication is the most important key to any leader's success; so to grow as leaders, you must learn how to be an effective communicator. No matter how powerful your message may be or how competent you are, if you can't clearly communicate, you will never reach your maximum level of leadership success.

'Ninety percent of leadership is the ability to communicate something people want.'

– Dianne Feinstein

Effective communication skills *(both verbal and non-verbal)* do not come naturally for most leaders. You need to practice *(both styles of communication)* repeatedly in order to become an excellent communicator. It may seem difficult to become an excellent communicator, but with practice, you'll soon discover that you can do it.

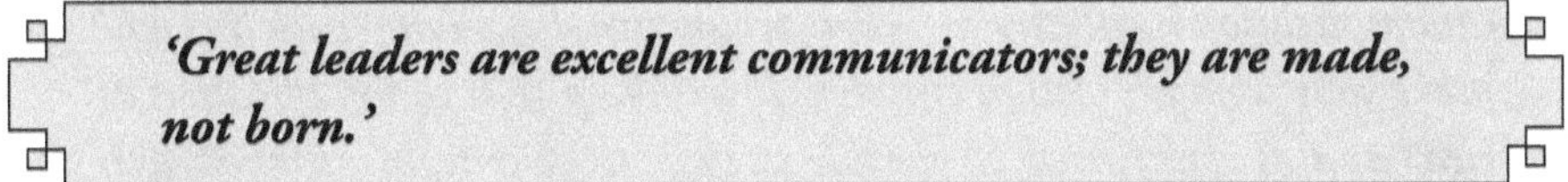

'Great leaders are excellent communicators; they are made, not born.'

In pharmaceutical selling, the biggest communication barrier is the difference of perception of the doctors and pharmaceutical sales people. Apart from verbal words, medical representatives should have good knowledge of body language, so that he can understand the signals conveyed by the doctor during the call. You have to spend more time on improving the communication skills of the medical representative and for these you must be an effective communicator that too in all round communication.

When you communicate effectively with your medical representatives it eliminates confusion and can foster a healthy and happy workplace. Effective communication with your medical representatives will also allow you to get work done more quickly and efficiently.

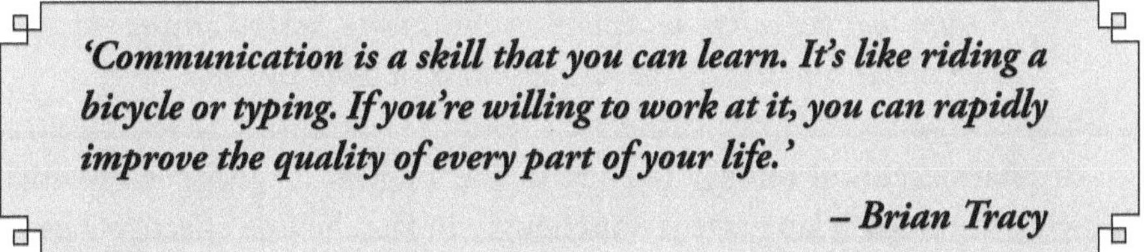

'Communication is a skill that you can learn. It's like riding a bicycle or typing. If you're willing to work at it, you can rapidly improve the quality of every part of your life.'

– Brian Tracy

VERBAL COMMUNICATION

Verbal communication is the use of sounds and words to express ourselves. This means sharing of information between individuals by using speech. An example of verbal communication is saying "No" when someone asks you to do something you don't want to do. It consists of only 7% of total communication because *'words are only carriers of the message, not the message.'* Verbal words cannot express the inner feeling of a person.

KEY POINTS: Verbal Communication

We communicate almost our entire day. We also make sure that our communication is effective as well as productive. Following check lists will make your communication effective. It will keep your communication as clear and as constructed as possible so that all your team members will have a full understanding of what you are saying.

1. *Words have the same effect as salt added to the food'; be careful about the choice of words as it plays an important role in communication. Poor selection of words can obstruct the understanding.*
2. *Be clear about your message. Always choose simple and right words.*
3. *Always keep your communication compact. Avoid lengthy communication because there is a possibility that the message may lost in the words. Remove all unnecessary words and stick to the point and keep it short and simple.*
4. *Use of terms like 'thank you' and 'please.'*
5. *Ensure that the communication shouldn't leave behind any doubt. The essence and style of the message must go hand in hand.*

In pharmaceutical selling, fluency in the English language is essential. Knowing the English language is not enough; in fact, how to effectively use it in communicating a thought precisely and tactfully is a skill that one has to learn.

IMPRESSIVE SPEAKING

Speaking is one of the most powerful things for a leader; use the right recipe and techniques and your speeches will forge motivated followers.

Speaking will have a sensational impact on your personal and professional life. Impressive speaking helps you to communicate the message precisely and effectively and is very important. When you speak impressively, you force medical representatives to listen to you. Impressive speaking and leadership qualities are closely linked. When leaders impressively speak, they simply do not pass the information; they actually communicate. First-line leaders who possess impressive speaking skills are able to influence and persuade medical representatives easily.

People do judge you by the way you speak!

English is a complicated language; here spelling does not determine the pronunciation. However, pronunciation is very crucial when it comes to effective communication. The words we use are greatly influenced by the quality of voice, the tone and the rhythm. When speaking, you have to control your tongue to produce the correct voice. We produce a lot of different sounds when we speak, and these sounds are often very different between one language and another. The words we use while speaking are a mixture of consonants and vowels. There are some general rules for pronouncing vowels and consonants. A vowel cannot be pronounced as a consonant. ***'A vowel needs a glide just as a consonant needs a sharp touch to the edge of the words.'*** Pleasant voices are articulated just when we appropriately utilise the blend of consonants and vowels. However, the voice is unique to the person to whom it belongs. For example, if confidence is low, it may be reflected by hesitancy in the voice; however, somebody who is confident will be more likely to have command of their voice and clarity of speech. Impressive speaking involves the following:

Projection of Voice: Projection is about being able to control the volume and the strength of your voice. An impressive voice should be clear and loud enough so that people can listen. For example, during presentation to a group, you need to ensure that you are heard even at the end of the room.

Articulation: Articulation is the movement of the tongue, lips, jaw and other speech organs in order to make a voice. There are many people who speak through clenched teeth and with little movement of their lips. It is their inability to open mouths and failure to make speech sounds with precision that is the root cause of inaudibility. The sound is locked into the mouth and not let out. To have good articulation it is important to unclench the jaw, open the mouth and give full benefit to each sound you make, paying particular attention to the ends of words.

Modulation: Modulation means varying the tone and pitch of your voice. Modulation makes the speech pleasant and interesting. Without modulation the speech becomes monotonous. Followings are the few component of modulation:

- **Speed** – This is the pace at which you talk. If speech is too fast then the audience will not have time to assimilate what is being said. Speaking at varying pace is a skill area and requires practice. You maintain your speed in such a way that the audience can understand what you are saying.
- **Pitch** – The pitch refers to how high and low you talk. Pitch depends on frequency of sound. Pitch of the voice changes with emotion. When we express anger, excitement or surprise the pitch will rise but while conveying sorrowful feelings the pitch will fall. Varying pitch is exceptionally vital to impact people.
- **Pause** – Pause means silence for a few seconds. Pauses are powerful. Pauses between words provide space for feeling and thinking. They can be used for effect to highlight the preceding statement or to gain attention before an important message.
- **Volume** – Volume is how loud a sound is, i.e. measure of sound. It is proportional to the amplitude of the sound wave. By raising or lowering volume occasionally, you can create emphasis.

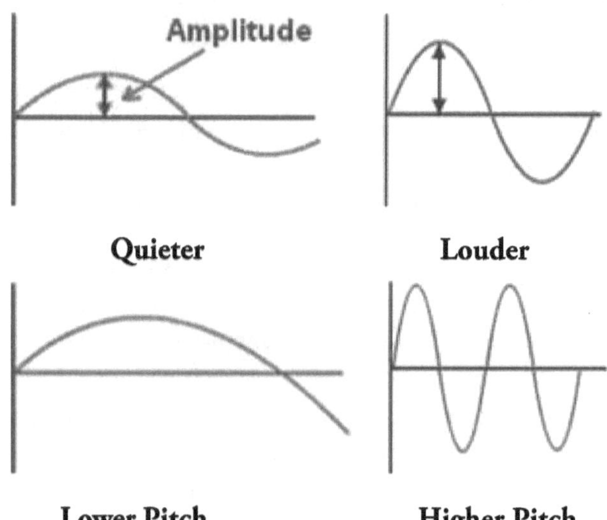

Your verbal message will only strengthen if you know how to present it correctly with the right voice.

KEY POINTS: Impressive Speaking

1. *Avoid monotone speech and highlight your words with vocal emphasis.*
2. *If you want your medical representatives to take notice of what you have to say, you'll need to consider how their ears are going to receive your message more than how you say to them.*
3. *Your passion and excitement force your medical representatives to listen to you.*
4. *Always move your mouth while talking. Your words should not be leaking through your lips because talking through your lips makes it difficult for others to understand.*
5. *Use appropriate tone as it acts as a highlighter on your words.*
6. *Maintain eye contact. Looking someone straight in the eye is the best way to influence others to listen to your words.*
7. *Impressive speaking requires that your words be heard and are well crafted and contains the message you intend to deliver.*

> ***'Good communication is just as stimulating as black coffee, and just as hard to sleep after.'***
>
> ***– Anne Morrow Lindbergh***

TONE OF VOICE

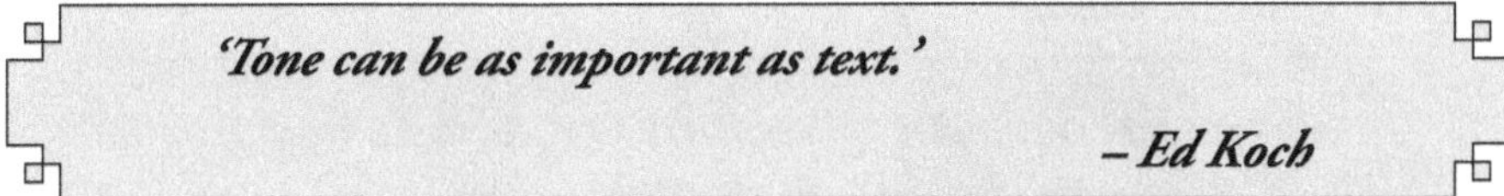

'Tone can be as important as text.'
– Ed Koch

The second key element of communicating a message is the tone of voice. Tone represents 38 percent of the message we are sending. Tone is a complex notion; it is not what you say, but how you say it. Tone is related to the way you convey your words, i.e., it is the expression of inner feelings. Tone of voice attracts or distracts the attention of people towards what you say. In fact, tone shows the mentality of the speaker as it can produce anger, guilt, sympathy or even love and romance. Tone includes the volume you use, the level and type of emotion that you convey. The same sentence can have various meanings depending on which tone you use.

For example: "come here, Simran."

You can say the above phrase in different ways using the following tones:

- Commanding or bossy
- Loving
- Angry
- Excited

Tone of your voice can change the whole meaning of your words. The words we use to convey a message can be given additional attention by the tone of our voice.

Importance of tone

Since tone is an evidence of your attitude towards the audience, you must be careful and work upon improving your ability to use an appropriate tone. Knowing what tone is appropriate for your specific message is an art. Your tone of voice determines how your medical representatives respond to you. Researchers showed that 90% of the conflict arises due to wrong tone of voice and 10% is due to difference in opinion. Today's communication is dynamic in nature where a tone of voice that is more conversational rather than commanding will win you respects. Today's medical representatives respond to conversation rather than command. You need to vary your tone of voice to fit the situation.

In our context, majority of conflicts are due to wrong tone of voice. Change the tone and see the change. Proper tone does not eliminate conflict but turn it to constructive or positive ends.

NON-VERBAL COMMUNICATION

Non-verbal communication is defined as the communication without words. In this kind of communication, we express our feelings, emotions, attitudes, opinions through our body movements. Charlie Chaplin, the famous silent movie actor was the pioneer of non-verbal communication; he was the only means of communication available on the screen. Our thoughts are accompanied by different body movements. As ***'action speaks louder than words'***; so non-verbal communication is extremely influential in interpersonal relationships.

The variance between the actual words of people and your understanding of what they are communicating comes from non-verbal communication, also referred to as Body Language. Body Language speaks the fact, which is not audible and it adds a new dimension to human communication. It represents 55 percent of our total communication and can make the difference.

'The language of the body is the key that can unlock the soul.'

Body language is considered the most important aspect of communication as it sends signals to how we are truly feeling. Body language demonstrates attitude. Just as tone, changes in our body language will change the meaning of the overall message we convey.

Being a first-line leader you should learn how to interpret the body language of your internal and external customers. Always look at the non-verbal signals to reinforce your interpretation. Body movements explain you the things that people cannot, will not or do not wish to say. Understanding body movements helps you to communicate more effectively. Body language, a subset of non-verbal communication, supplements verbal communication in social interaction. Body language comprises of followings –

1. Eye Contact
2. Facial Expression
3. Postures
4. Gestures

1. Eye Contact

> ***'It's hard to hold a conversation with people when you're not seeing them.'***
>
> ***– Dale Ludwig***

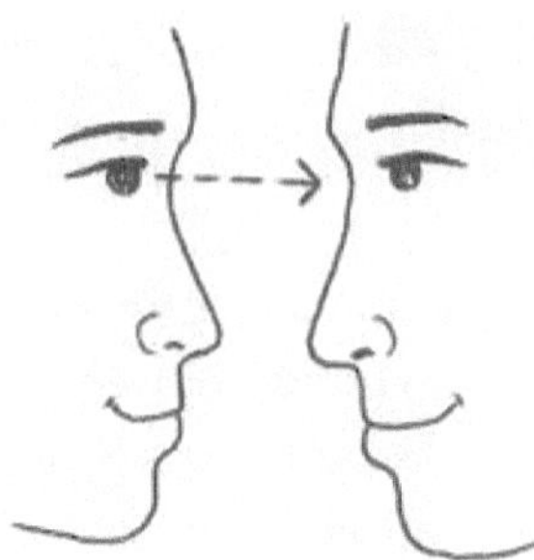

The eyes are the most expressive part of the human body. Perhaps, eyes are the best and easiest way to judge a person. Eyes are called *'the windows to our soul'* and *'mirror of our heart.'* Eye contact refers to two individuals looking into each other's eyes at the same time.

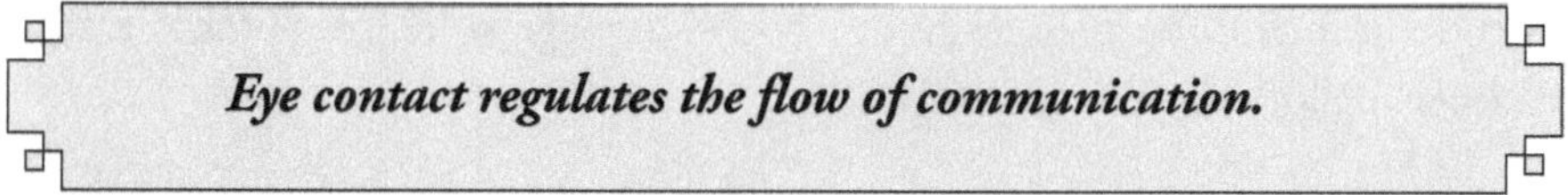

Eye contact regulates the flow of communication.

Eye contact is an incredibly expressive form of non-verbal communication. The objective is to make other people (whom you are communicating with) feel comfortable; for example; if they look at you, look at them and if they look away; you look away. Always pause for a few seconds before looking at the eyes.

Eye contact between two persons is a powerful act of communication and may show interest, affection or dominance. The directions in which eyes move indicates whether the person is hearing, visualising or feeling. For example:

Looking Upward

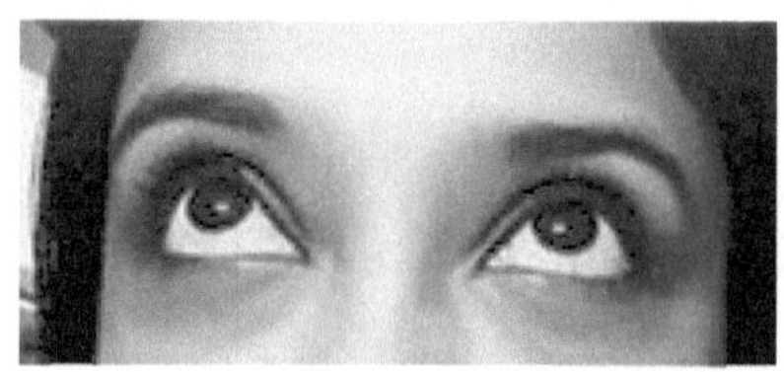

Often implies thinking, making pictures in the head indicates a visual thinker. We look up to the left when we remember images from the past and we look up to the right when constructing a mental picture from words.

Looking Downward

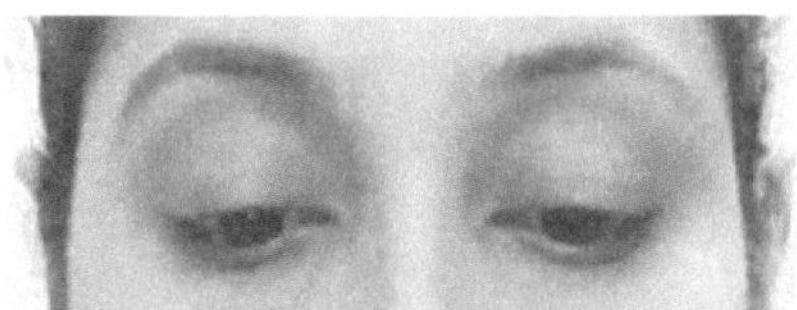

A sign of submission, it can also demonstrate that the individual is feeling guilty.

Glancing

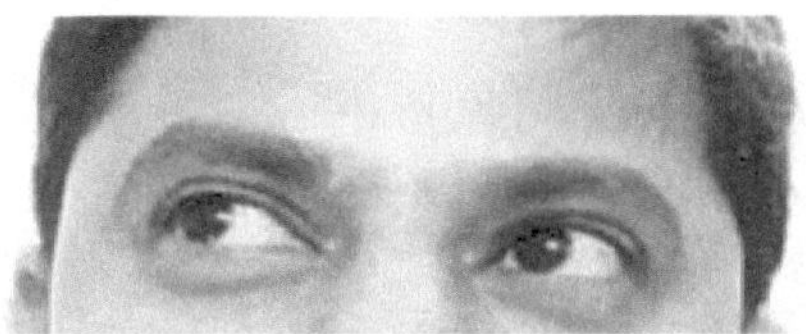

Glance means a quick and short look. Glancing at a person can show a desire to talk with them. Glancing sideways at a person with raised eyebrows can be an indication of interest. Without the raised eyebrow it will probably be disappointing.

Making eye contact – Looking at a person recognises them and shows that you are interested in them, especially if you look in their eyes. If a person says something when you are turning away and afterward you make eye contact, then this indicates they have snatched your attention.

Breaking eye contact – Breaking eye contact can demonstrate that something that has recently been said that makes individuals not have any desire to maintain eye contact.

Long eye contact – Eye contact longer than normal can have a few distinct implications.

Limited eye contact – When people make very little eye contact, they may be feeling uncertain.

Blinking

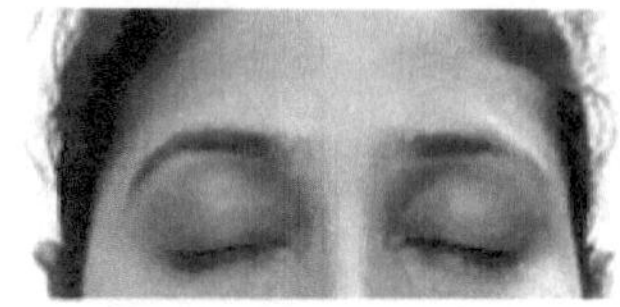

Blinking is a neat natural process whereby the eyelids wipe the eyes clean, much as a windscreen wiper on a car.

Winking

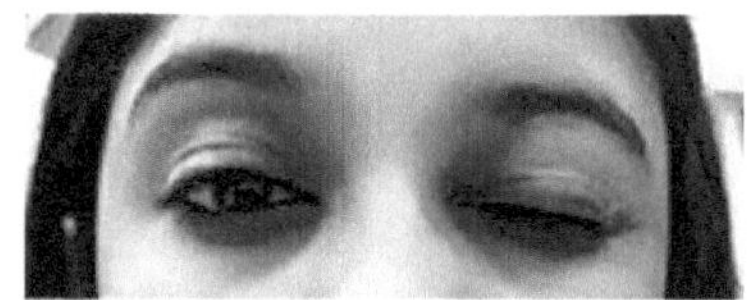

Closing one eye in a wink is a signal that typically recommends conspiratorial ('you and I both understand, though others do not').

Tears – Actual tears that move down the cheeks are often a symptom of extreme fear or bitterness, although incomprehensibly you can also weep tears of joy.

KEY POINTS: Eye Contact

1. *Eye contact shows your interest to whom, you are talking.*
2. *It allows you to receive non-verbal signals from the audience.*
3. *You can gauge the impact of your remarks.*
4. *You can detect the level of understanding in the listeners.*
5. *It enhances your credibility.*
6. *During a two-way conversation, people look each other for 30 to 60 percent.*
7. *Beyond 60 percent means more interested in the person than conversation.*
8. *Longer eye contact is required during listening.*
9. *Based on the emotional state, the size of the pupils changes.*
10. *People of different cultures have different eye contact.*

2. Facial Expression

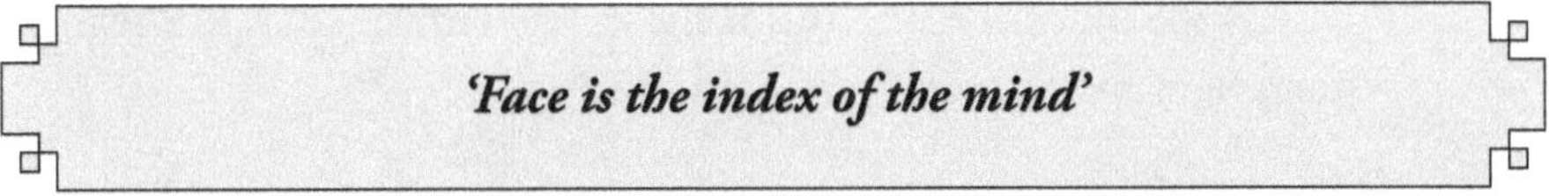

'Face is the index of the mind'

Facial expression is very important as it reflects the internal emotions through faces. Facial expression is a combination of smiling, reactions of eyebrows, the eye, the nose, the lips and the chin. The muscles of our faces are evolved as a system for signalling feelings and attitude. For example, when someone is happy or upset, it is clear through his or her face. It is obvious that people can forget the spoken words but they can remember the facial expressions. When you are communicating, you must be aware that your verbal communication matches your facial expression.

Smile

'The shortest distance between people is a smile.'

A smile is a happy expression on the face in which the ends of the mouth turn up. Smile is a global language which is understood, around the world. There is a saying that *'the most expensive dress in your wardrobe is a smile on your face.'* It not only shows interest but there is much more to it. For example; a smile associated with eye contact communicates greetings while a big/ broad smile communicates victory. Smiling also has an actual impact on your physiology, i.e. how you feel.

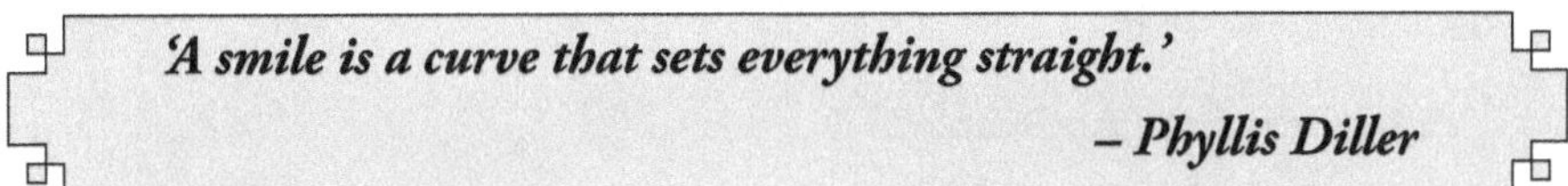

'A smile is a curve that sets everything straight.'

– Phyllis Diller

There are two types of smile:

1. **Honest Smile:**

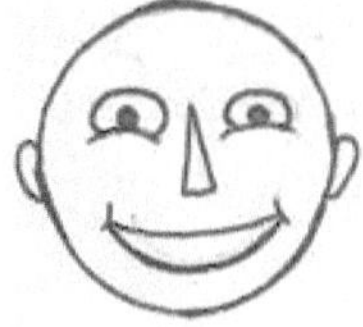

An honest smile involves the entire face including the eyes. More than just the mouth, numerous facial muscles are in action. The most noticeable is the tightening around the eyes.

2. **Artificial Smile:**

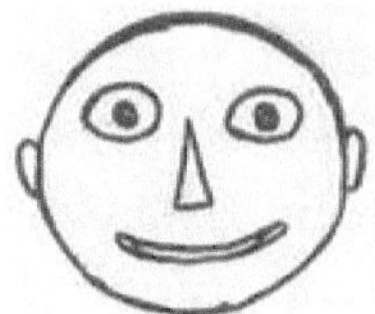

People who put on an artificial smile just utilise the muscles around the mouth. But the upper part of their face remains virtually unchanged. Their smile is also less likely to be showing their teeth. This smile could mean the person is not telling every bit of relevant information.

There is a physiological distinction between an honest and artificial smile: two muscles are involved *(zygomatic major and orbicularis oculi).* Honest smiles involve both muscles and artificial smiles the former but not the latter. An honest smile is typically one that involves not just the eyes, but the skin around the eyes and the formation of crow's feet. When someone's giving you an artificial smile, they often concentrate too much on what their mouth is doing, and you'll be able to see a larger number of teeth than you would during an honest smile.

3. Postures

Postures reflects personality

Postures specify how you position your body. Posture has great significance in interpreting body language as it can amplify or nullify the words you speak. Unlike facial expressions, postures observed or detected from long distance thus it has the power to convey a message to many. Posture is a matter of habit as it reflects your intentions. For example, people with bent shoulders are perceived as lazy, passive and indecisive compared to people who hold themselves straight with open shoulders and hands-on-hips.

Correct Postures

- It gives you strengths and projects you as a confident person.
- Head held high in neutral position with the ears in line with the shoulder line.
- The shoulders are resting down. Your chest should be open.
- Feet are firmly on the ground, distributing the weight evenly between both heels.
- You should have a very minor strain in your abdomen and buttocks muscles to keep your composure.

Inappropriate postures can be insulting or annoying.

Postures can indicate not only how people feel but also how they view situations. While communicating with customers, if you stand straight with your chin raised, arms relaxed and hanging down at your sides, it indicates your confidence. On the other hand, your body is stiff and your hands are clasped firmly in front of him, it indicates lack of confidence.

4. Gestures

Gesture conveys emotion

Gestures include purposeful movement of the hands, face, or other parts of the body. A gesture is a form of non-verbal communication in which visible bodily actions communicate particular messages, either in place of, or in conjunction with speech. Gestures are used to clarify or emphasise ideas and thus strengthen verbal communication. Gestures may be voluntary or involuntary. Gestures can be classified into two groups:

- **Speech Independent** – A wave or a V for a peace sign are examples of speech independent gestures.
- **Speech Related** – This is required to give supplemental information to a verbal message; for example, pointing to an object for discussion.

KEY POINTS: Gestures

1. *Gestures are spontaneous and depend upon the situation.*
2. *When you approach a customer, your gestures create your first impression. To interact with your customer in a better way, you must learn to interpret their gestures.*
3. *When first-line leaders don't use gestures correctly, it recommends they don't perceive the critical issues, they have no passionate interest in the issues or they don't understand the effect of their non-verbal conduct on the medical representatives.*
4. *To use gestures effectively, you must be aware of how those movements will most likely be perceived.*
5. *In order to be effective, you must control your gestures.*

Like spoken language, gestures also differ from culture to culture and place to place. Many gestures have different interpretations across the globe. Here are some common gestures and the messages behind them:

Hand Gestures

Gestures of hands have been studied in-depth and the interpretations are undoubtedly very interesting. The expression of your face also changes when you use your hands for the purpose of communication. Hand gestures often signify the state of well-being of the person. Relaxed hands express confidence and self-assurance, while clenched hands may be understood as signs of anxiety or anger. If a person is wringing his/her hands, this demonstrates nervousness. Followings are the common hand gestures:

Rubbing the palms – Usually, rubbing the palms together is a manner in which a person conveys positive expectations. For example, a magician often rubs his palms with a hope of something positive.

Hand on heart – This gesture usually conveys a person's desire to be believed or accepted. This gesture also indicates greeting other people, swearing an oath etc.

Hand in the pocket – This indicates both the authority and casual approach of the person. Hand in pocket creates a negative impression.

Clenched fist – Clenched fist with thumbs tucked-in indicates inconvenience. The person is anxious and trying to get a grip on himself. *'You cannot shake hands with a clenched fist.'*

Chopping movements – Chopping is for attention, and is normally authoritative. A person who *"chops'* has decided and is not probably going to change it.

Palm Gestures

Human palms convey powerful non-verbal signals. There are three palm gestures:

a) **Palm up** – When the palm facing upward also called submissive palm position indicates that a person may be asking something as in the case of a beggar.

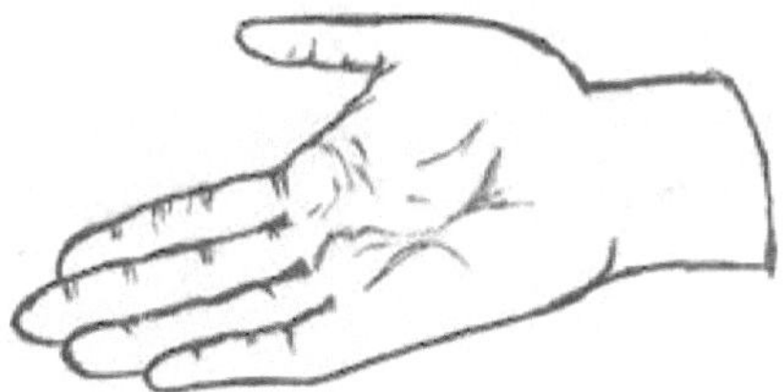

b) **Palm down** – When the palm facing downwards, also called dominant palm position indicates authority and only acceptable in cases where the person to whom you give the request is your subordinate.

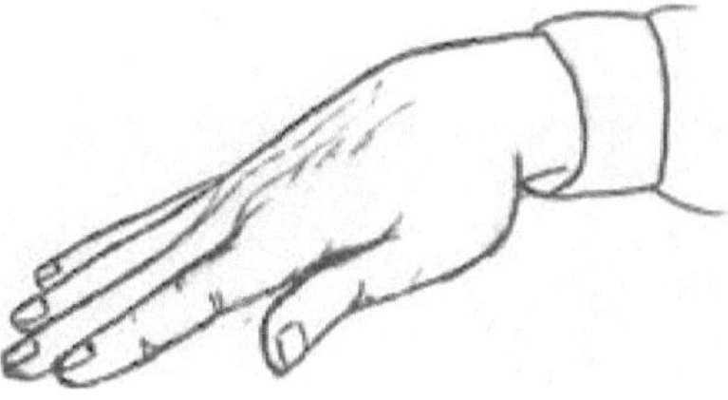

c) **Palm closed finger pointed** – The palm is closed into a fist with a pointed finger, also called aggressive palm position indicates that the speaker compels his listener into submission. The pointed finger is one of the most irritating and annoying gestures that a person can use while speaking, particularly when it beats time to the speaker's words.

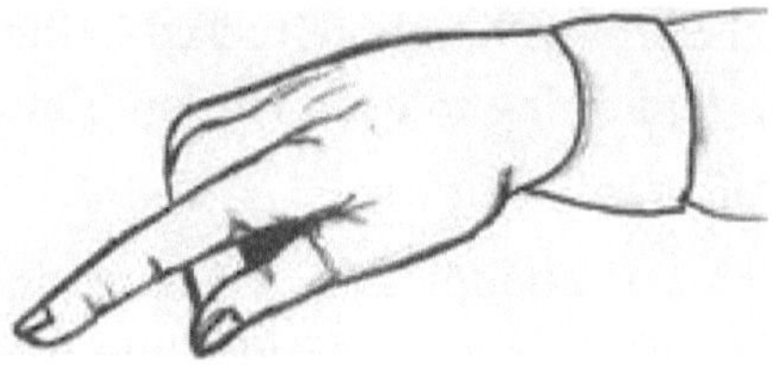

d) **Thumbs up**

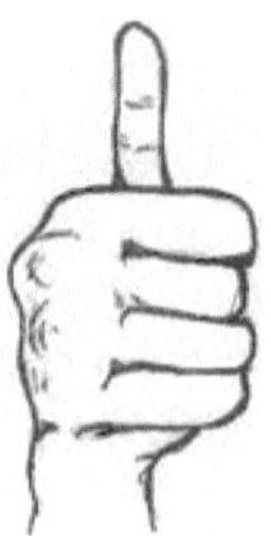

In India, thumbs up communicates OK, however if the thumb is jerked sharply upwards it indicates an insult meaning 'sit on this!' These gestures have different interpretations across the globe, for example in some countries it is regarded as an insult.

Ring or Ok gesture

Here the thumb and forefinger make a circle. In all English speaking countries, the ring or OK gestures stands for "All correct." It means well done or top class. However, in a few countries, there are different views about this gesture. In Japan, it means money while in France it is zero.

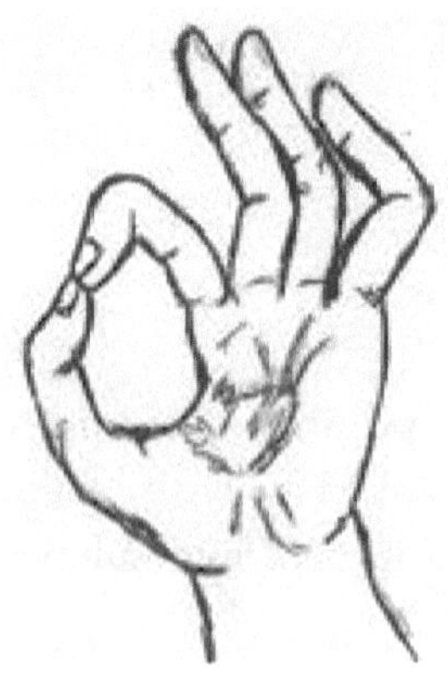

Fingers in the mouth

The fingers are placed in the mouth when a person is under pressure; by doing this the person tries to relieve stress.

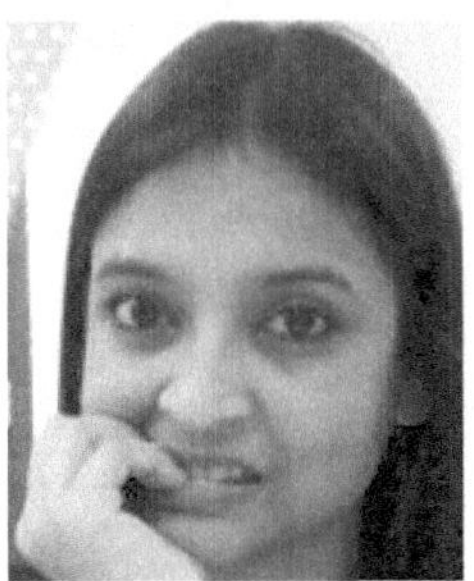

Head nodding

Head nodding gesture normally implies agreement or bowing, a surrendered signal that shows one is obliging with another person's opinions.

Lowered head

Lowered head implies that one is hiding something. When you bring down your head while you are being complimented, you may be displaying shyness, disgrace, or timidity. It may also convey that you are keeping distance from another person, showing disbelief, or contemplating internally.

Forgetfulness

The slapping of the head demonstrates forgetfulness.

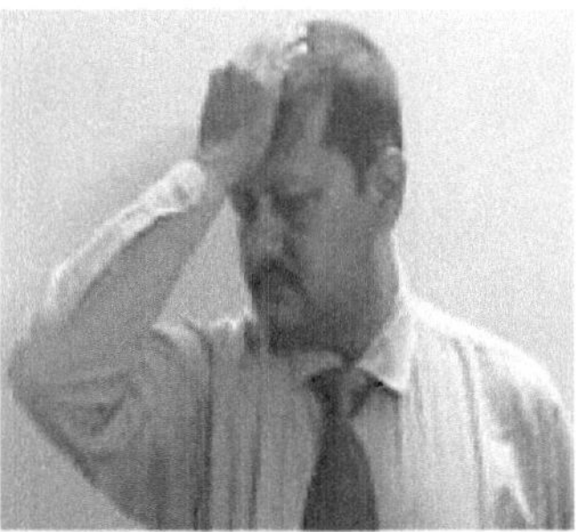

Head Gestures

Human head can also send a wide range of signals. There are two main head gestures:

- **Neutral Head Position** – The position taken by the person who has an unbiased attitude about what he is hearing. The head typically stays still and may occasionally give small nods.

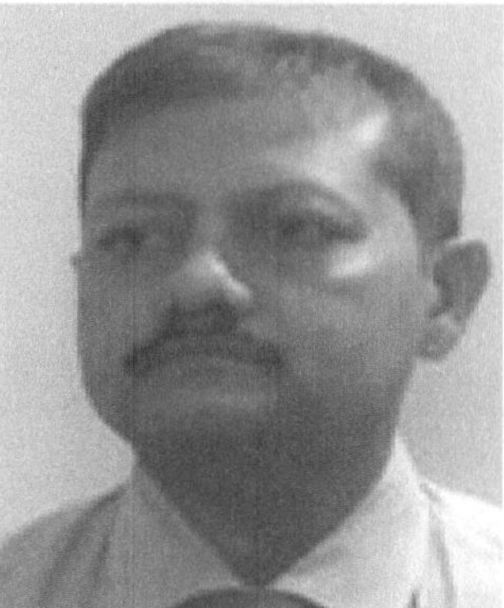

- **Interested Head Position** – When the head inclines to one side it shows that interest has been created.

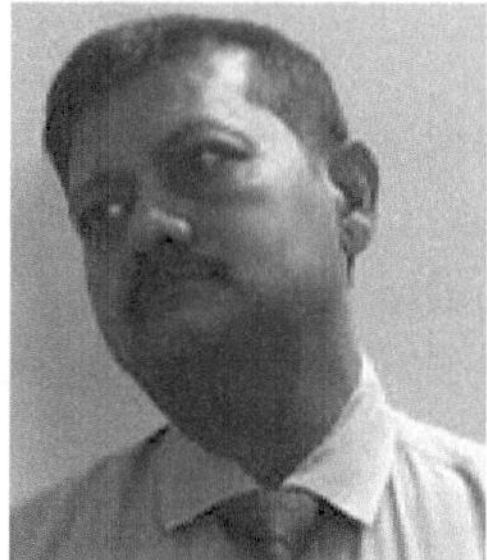

Both Hands Behind Head

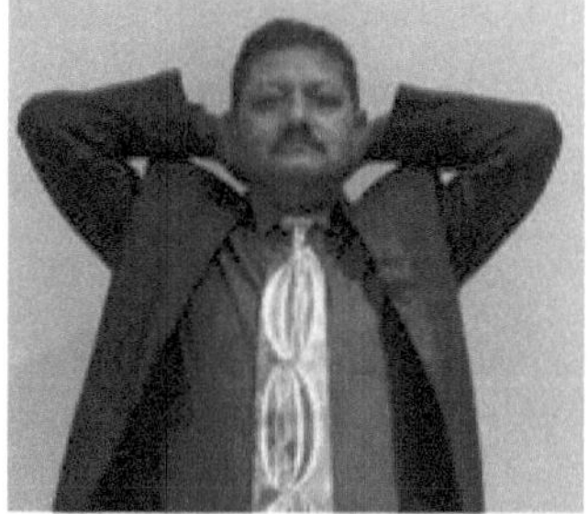

This gesture is usually displayed by the people who are feeling confident, dominant, or superior about something. This gesture communicates that everything is under control.

PHYSICAL CONTACT – TOUCH

Physical contact or touch is a very powerful non-verbal communication. Physical contact is secret behind many successful relationships. A touch can say a lot of words. This is likely most evident when somebody you know is in an unfortunate situation or in distress, taking hold of his or her hand or putting an arm around the shoulder often is considerably more effective than words.

Different touches convey different messages. For example; a handshake is professional, a push to someone is threatening. There are many opportunities to communicate through touch, without requiring verbal clarification. Additional alert must be taken when communicating through touch in different cultures, and there are definite boundaries depending upon the social standard. For example, in country like India, be extremely cautious while making a touch with someone of the opposite gender.

You should know the effectiveness of using touch while communicating to your medical representatives.

> ***'If a word of praise is accompanied by a touch on the shoulder, that's the gold star on the ribbon.'***
>
> ***– D. Walton***

HANDSHAKE

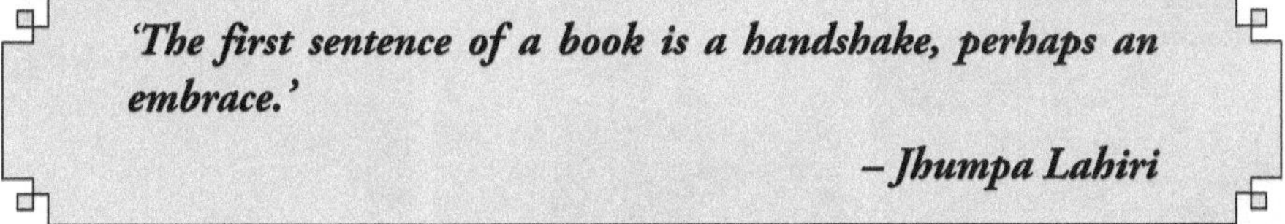

> ***'The first sentence of a book is a handshake, perhaps an embrace.'***
>
> ***– Jhumpa Lahiri***

Handshake is a very common an essential type of gesture used very often in the business world. Since a handshake is the first contact made between two individuals, it is essential that it be executed accurately to build up a positive first impression. The way one shakes hands provides us with a signal about his/her personality. For instance, an aggressive person uses firm grip whereas a person with low self-esteem normally has a soft handshake. The handshake is commonly used both during the initial welcome and while leaving. Following are the important points of a good handshake

- Make eye contact
- Smile
- Extend your right hand
- Lean forward
- Firmly grasp
- Shake hands for two or three times
- After second or third shake, release
- Be confident

There are three aspects of handshakes; dominance, submission and equality:

Dominance is conveyed when your palm faces down in the handshake. Dominance implies that the person wants to take control of the encounter.

When your palm faces up, it means submission. This is just the opposite of dominance.

When the palms are in a vertical position it shows mutual respect and a feeling of equality. This position transmits a feeling of respect towards the other.

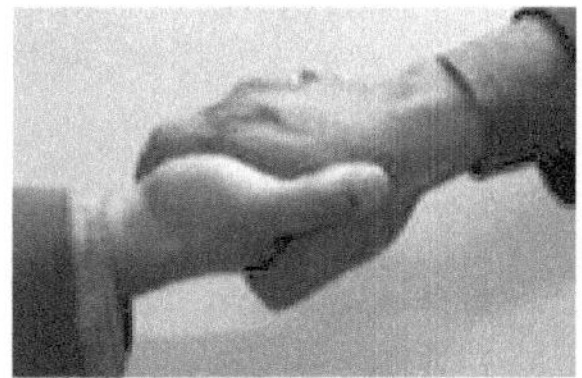

Dominance
Taking the Control

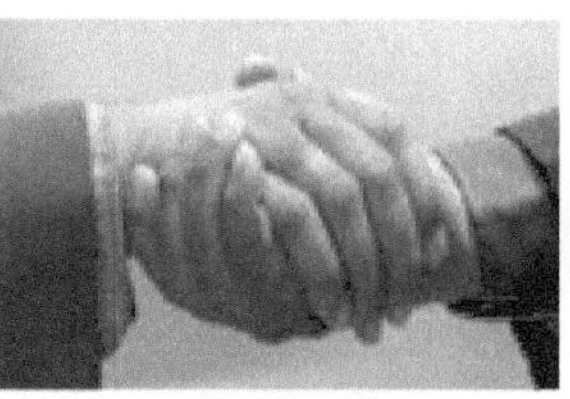

Submission
Giving the Control

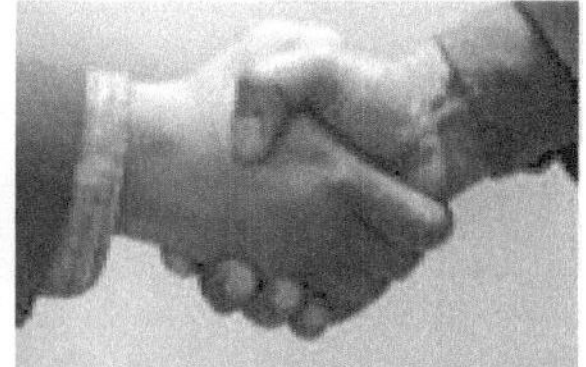

Equality
Actual Shaking

Glove Handshake – In this position, one person puts his left hand on top of the normal handshake thereby trapping the other person's hand. The initiator tries to give the receiver the feeling that he/she is trustworthy and genuine. When a glove handshake is used in a meeting with a person for the first time, it may have a negative impact. The receiver feels suspicious and cautious about the initiator's intentions. This kind of handshake should be used with only known people.

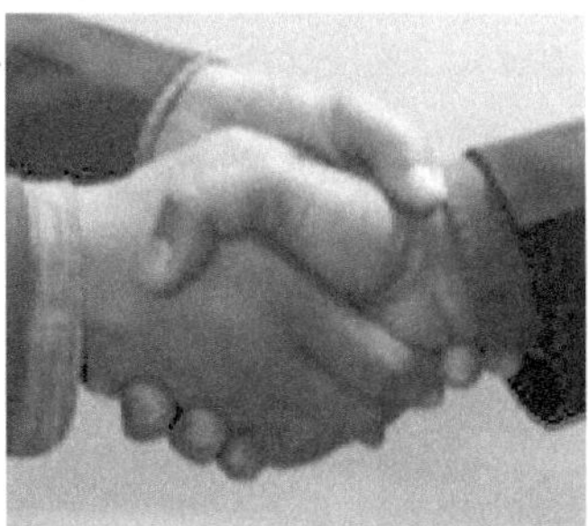

Body language is an excellent subject. There are many books available on body language. I suggest you read to strengthen your understanding further. I have tried to provide a few tips above that will give you an idea about its importance in our professional lives. You can improve your communication skills when you understand the meaning of different postures and gestures, taking into account cultural differences.

PROXEMICS

Proxemics is the study of how people utilise space when they are communicating. The space and orientation (how people face towards or away from each other) between people during interaction express much about how they like each other and the relationship between them. For example, we stand closer to people and turn our body in their direction when we certainly biased towards them. Basically there are four kinds of spaces that people generally use in communication. This can vary by place and different cultures and have diverse guidelines.

The four kinds of spaces are –

Intimate Zone	**Personal Zone**	**Social Zone**	**Public Zone**
0 to 18 Inches	18 inches to 4 feet	4 to 12 feet	above 12 feet
People emotionally close to you, are allowed to enter in this zone	The distance you would stand during friendly gathering	The distance you would stand with someone you don't know well	The distance you feel comfortable when addressing a big group

1. **Intimate Zone** – This is up to 18 inches from your body. This is for people who you are very close to you. Only those who are emotionally close such as parents, spouse, children etc. are allowed to enter. People in intimate zones share a unique level of comfort with one another. Exceptional circumstances like contact sports, public transport are allowed in the intimate zone.

2. **Personal Zone** – This zone is 18 inches to 4 feet. This is reserved for talking to friends or family. You stand at this distance from the peers of your office, your superiors, your subordinates or your customers. Personal zone is close to the intimate zone and may involve touching. When an outsider approaches someone in the personal zone he or she is likely to feel uncomfortable or awkward.

3. **Social Zone** – It is about 4 to 12 feet. More formal social and business interaction occur in this zone. In a social zone touching is not possible; however, a handshake can be made only when both the persons stretch out their hand in order to bridge the gap. You stand in this zone from people, whom you do not know very well.

4. **Public Zone** – This zone starts from 12 feet and may extend to 30 feet or to the range of eyesight and bearing. Whenever you address a large group of people, this is a comfortable distance you choose to stand. For example; if you are at an event listening to a professor giving a lecture, you are probably about 12 to 25 feet away.

LISTENING

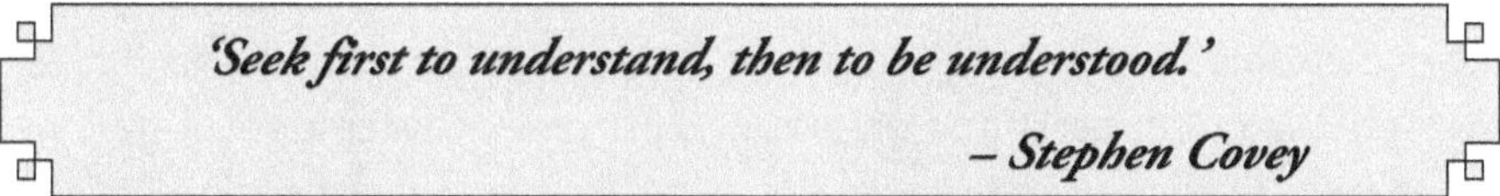

'Seek first to understand, then to be understood.'

– Stephen Covey

Effective leaders are magnificent communicators. Listening is the foundation of effective communication. Out of four communication modes (i.e. speaking, writing, reading and listening), listening represents 40% to 50% of our communications and it requires more intelligence than speaking. We may hear but we may not listen. Listening is not just hearing as it involves both ear and brain. During hearing, sound waves strike the eardrum, causing vibrations which are transmitted to the brain. Listening occurs only when the brain swings into action by reconstructing these electrochemical impulses by giving meaning to the sounds.

KEY POINTS: Listening

1. *People respond to those who listen to them.*
2. *Listening is the single best way to learn what is going on.*
3. *Listen in such a way that others love to speak to you.*
4. *Effective listening is a challenging work.*
5. *Developing listening skill needs practice.*

Active Listening

'Active listening' implies, as its name proposes, actively listening. It is an ability that can be obtained and developed with practice. However, active listening can be difficult to master and will, therefore, require significant investment and persistence to develop. Active listening is also about patience – pauses and short periods of silence to be acknowledged. Active listening includes giving the other individual time to explore their thoughts and feelings, they should, therefore, be given satisfactory time for that.

Empathetic Listening

Listening empathically means to listen with the purpose to see how the speaker feels in addition to understanding his or her thoughts. Empathetic listening is the highest form of listening because we listen not only through ears but also through our mind, heart and emotions. This type of listening will motivate the speaker to share more openly his ideas, feelings etc. Empathic listening is required when there is an issue that needs resolving, or if there is conflict present. Allow the expression of feelings and sharing of problems.

Key Points: Empathetic Listening

1. *Have a proper eye contact and body language.*
2. *Be ready, attentive to the speaker.*
3. *Create a positive atmosphere.*
4. *Reflect your comprehension back to the speaker*
5. *Use appropriate tone of your voice.*

According to Peter Drucker, '60% of all management problems are the result of faulty communication.' In fact, the majority of communication problems come from poor listening. The big miss for most first-line leaders is that they fail to understand that the purpose of communication is not to message, but to engage and this requires listening. If you want to be a better first-line leader, talk less and listen more.

Following are techniques to improve the listening skill –

Stop talking – During listening stop talking to others, even to yourself.

Paying complete attention – When you are really listening to someone, imagine that only two people exist. Always sit with your back straight, this improves your attentiveness. Face the speaker directly, lean forward and pay complete attention.

Develop eye contact – Listening is an art. Listen with your eyes also. Always look at the speaker while listening, this is an assurance that you are listening. Raising an eyebrow slightly if something sparks interest.

Showing that you are listening – Smile or nod occasionally. Support the speaker with verbal comments like 'I see,' 'hmms' etc. to show that you understand and are willing to continue listening.

Keeping an open mind – Listen carefully. Clear your mind and focus on what the speaker is saying.

Listen without interruption – Whenever someone wants to talk to you, listen single-mindedly without interruption. Interrupting can send the wrong message. Wait for the speaker to complete what he/she wants to say.

Paying attention to what is not being said 'Non-Verbal Hints' – The key to be an excellent listener is listening not only for the words but for what is going on behind the words. While listening, look at the body movements. Listen for the actual message and focus your attention on the speaker.

Ask questions for clarification – Asking questions is a technique that confirms that you were truly listening to what the other person was saying. Never assume that you completely understand what the speaker really said or meant. Instead, ask questions like 'how do you feel about that?' or 'how do you mean?' The best way is to paraphrase what the speaker has said (what you have been listening to) and repeat it back to the speaker so that the speaker can clarify you if required. Asking questions is a process that gives you an opportunity to listen more and sell more.

Feed it back – This is a technique to prove that you were actually listening. Here you can say like 'what you really mean is that? Is this correct? When you do this or feed it back to the speaker in your own words, you prove to them that you were really listening to the speaker because you value them and what they have to say.

Take a note – You must take notes while listening to your team members. These notes not only help you to understand but also give you an opportunity to assess the points later.

> ***'If you spend more time asking appropriate questions rather than giving answer or opinions, your listening skills will increase.'***
>
> ***– Brain Koslow***

Replace bad listening habits with good listening techniques!

SITUATION

When medical representative doesn't listen and tries to dominate conversation

Medical representatives sometimes intend not to listen or to take over the conversations. The probable reason may be their own enthusiasm, ideas, disagreement or priorities seem so important. Whatever be the reason, the medical representative who doesn't listen is difficult to work with. This will cost the organisation and as a leader you have to deal with the consequences. Before taking corrective measures try to identify the followings:

1. *Is the inability to listen a recent development or a chronic habit?*
2. *Why this medical representative not listen?*
3. *Is he aware of his poor listening?*
4. *Have you even given feedback about this?*

The answers of the above will determine the method you choose to explore him. In case the medical representative is unaware and would be willing to try and correct it, recommend some skill training followed by individual coaching. If the inability to listen is from arrogance, then you have to take a blunt approach with some recommendations of skills training.

Be patient, speak specifically about your observations and do not let any misunderstanding develop. You have to stay focused and keep yourself calm.

It is very difficult to talk to someone who won't or can't listen and it takes multiple sessions to improve.

Give constructive feedback as often as possible. Remember listening well is not easy; it needs practice and dedication to improve. Offer your support and demonstrate good listening skills consistently.

COMMUNICATION STYLES

We all are communicators. Whether we are writing, speaking or listening, we are continuously expressing our thoughts, feelings and ideas. A communication style is the way we share information with others. How well our messages come across can depend on the style of communication we use. Good communication skills require a high level of self-awareness. Being aware of your own communication style can help you to understand how your communication is perceived by others. By becoming more aware of how others see you, you can adjust promptly to their styles of communicating. People feel great when the other person speaks with them in their own particular styles. There are three basic communication styles:

1. Offensive

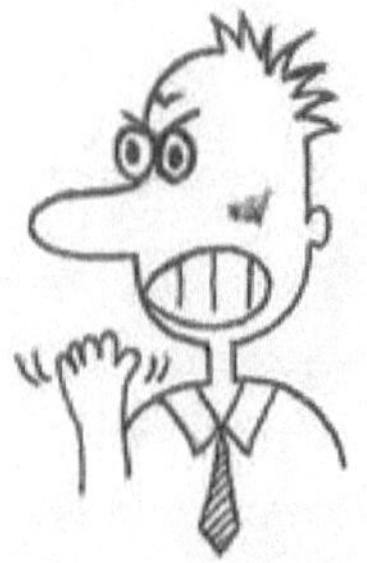

'I am ok, You're not'

Offensiveness is defined by a lack of respect for others. This is a harmful style and can end up worsening social anxiety by making others view you more harshly. The characteristics of this style are:

- Superiority is maintained by putting others down.
- People often feel crushed by an encounter with an offensive person.
- You stand up for your personal rights and express your thoughts, feelings and beliefs in a way that violates the rights of the other person.

2. Submissive

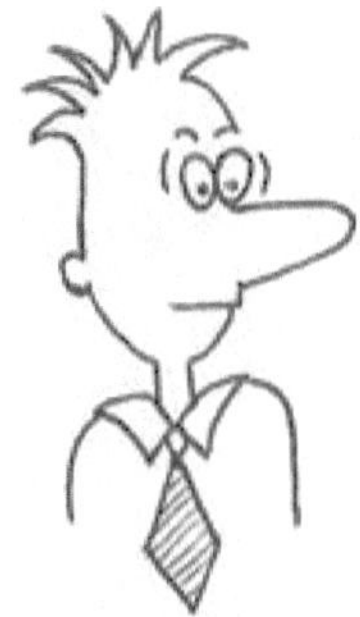

'You are ok, I am not'

Submissiveness is defined by a lack of respect for one's self. It is ineffective style of communication where the sender is unable to convey his thoughts or views out of fear of confrontation by others. The characteristics are:

- Not expressing honest feelings, thoughts and beliefs.
- Allowing others to violate your rights.
- Violating your own rights.

3. Assertive

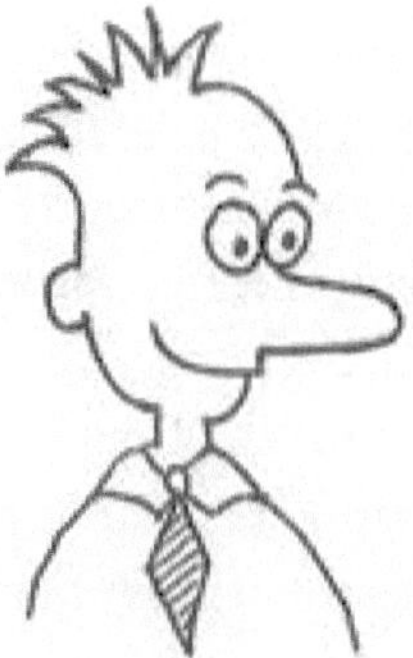

'I am ok, you are also ok.'

It is the effective style of communication, where you communicate your needs, feelings, opinions, and beliefs in an open and honest manner without violating the rights of others. This style is based on mutual respect. Assertive people strike a right balance of respect for other's opinions while stating their needs and wants in a way that cannot be misinterpreted.

Benefits of being assertive

Assertiveness means to have respect and being assertive will make you feel valued, understood, and important to the people around you. Being assertive will:

- Help you become self-confident.
- Increases self-esteem.
- Earn respect from others.
- Improves your communication skills.
- Improve your decision-making ability.

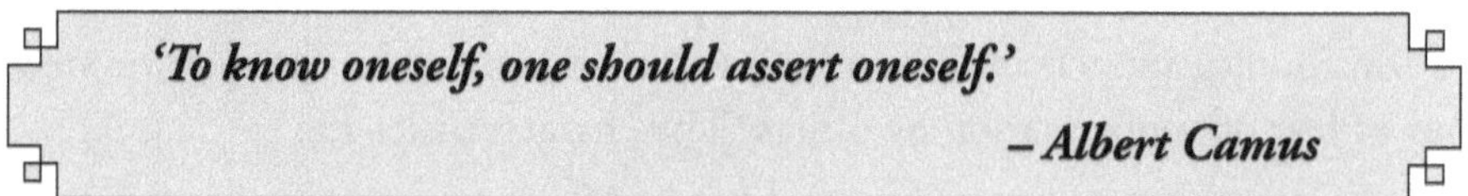

'To know oneself, one should assert oneself.'
– Albert Camus

First-line leaders need to be assertive

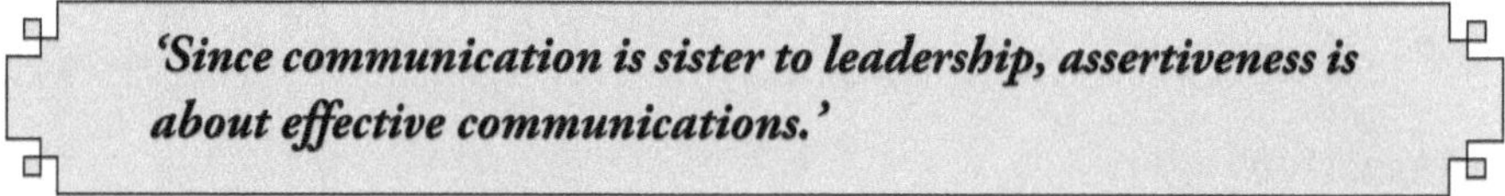

'Since communication is sister to leadership, assertiveness is about effective communications.'

Assertiveness is the capacity to express your thoughts and feelings in such a way that clearly states your needs and keeps the lines of communication open with the other. Effective communication and strong interpersonal relationships are essential to good leadership, and there are situations where the assertive style option will obtain better results. The way you communicate will have a big impact on how you get on with medical representatives and get the things you want. Being assertive will confirm that you respect yourself and your medical representatives. Being assertive is not easy; like any other skills, assertiveness can be learned. You have to commit to it and practise until you are confident with your ability to stand up for yourself. *'Leaders were not born Assertive.'*

KEY POINTS: Assertiveness

1. *Be genuine and direct about your feelings, needs and convictions.*
2. *Sate your views without being apologetic.*
3. *Learn to say 'No' to unreasonable expectations.*
4. *Recognise and respect the rights of others.*
5. *Be aware of body language and maintain eye contact.*

Chapter 6

LEADERSHIP STYLES

> ***'Different people require different leadership styles at different times in their career.'***

The objective of a leader, on a general note, is to get things done (by others) by making optimum use of available resources. How leaders manage always depends on their leadership style and personality. Some leaders follow the organisation's systems and do not use their discretion, some leaders are inclined to bring about changes and regularly apply their discretion, whereas some leaders possess magnetic personality etc. They all try to adhere to the organisation's mission as well as objectives. Leaders adopt different styles to accomplish the team's objectives. Most of us have encountered the various types of leaders. Leaders are mostly typecast according to the different types of leadership styles, personality, function and involvement. Followings are different leadership style –

- Autocratic
- Laissez-Faire
- Bureaucratic
- Democratic
- Coercive
- Transactional
- Transformational

Autocratic – This style also known as Authoritarian Style which can be described as *'My way or the highway.'* Leader is the decision-making authority and focuses on control. Leaders tell their team what is to be done and how it is to be done, without asking for their inputs. Team members are expected to obey orders without explanations. This kind of style is only effective in companies where the type of work requires quick decision- making. The sole responsibility of the decision and the outcome is with the leader. Autocratic style works best when your team is inexperienced. For example, this style is required for newly joined medical representatives, and also when time is constrained for making a decision.

Autocratic style has some limitations. When members of the team are not involved in the decision-making process, they feel that they are not being considered as a part of the organisations, and this creates demotivations. This style creates a climate of fear because the team members are forced to follow the directions given by the leader. Team members get no opportunity for their development.

Laissez-Faire – Laissez-faire a French phrase means, 'let do.' This style is also known as delegative style and is direct opposite of the autocratic style. Leaders give team members as much freedom as possible. They delegate the work to their team depending on their skills and the team determines goals, makes decisions, and resolves problems on their own. Leaders support their team whenever required. This style is helpful when the team is highly skilled, experienced, and educated; and also the team has to be trustworthy and experienced. The Laissez-Faire style motivates the team members, boosts their confidence and allows them to learn how to be a leader themselves. This style promotes a climate of trust.

This style also has some limitations. If the team members lack sufficient skills, experience or motivation to complete the task, the organisation will suffer. In some cases, the team takes advantage of their powers for their own interest which may lead to disputes in the team. Also, the absence of proper supervision may result in poor productivity.

Bureaucratic – The leader manages *'by the book,' i.e.* Bureaucratic leaders rely on rules and regulations and clearly defined positions within organisations. According to them everything must be done as per the procedure or policy. If it isn't covered by the book, they refer to the next level above. This style is required to perform routine tasks.

This style allows organisations to manage people who do repetitive tasks. This style of leadership has no space to explore new ways to solve problems. This style is ineffective in teams and organisations that rely on flexibility, creativity or innovation.

Democratic – It is also referred to as participative style. This style is based on 'majority rule' where the leader allows team members to participate in the decision-making process. However, the final decision rests in the hands of the leader. This style is based on mutual respect. The team members get an opportunity to provide their thoughts and can evaluate their own performance. Everyone gets motivation as they are involved in the decision-making process. The democratic styles help to build relationships among the team members. Democratic styles provide opportunities for team members to develop a high sense of personal growth and job satisfaction.

The main drawback of this style is that the leaders can become overly dependent on the expertise and experience of their team. However, this style takes more time in decision-making as more and more members take part in it.

Coercive – This kind of style is like a power from a person's authority to punish. This kind of power is the capacity of a leader to force a team member to follow an order by warning him/her with punishment if he/she doesn't comply with the order. Good leaders use coercive power only as a last resort. This style is required for short term goals and when there is no other option. For instance, if an organisation is experiencing difficulty with employees using unsafe work practices, the leader might utilise the coercive style to gain immediate compliance with the organisation's safety standards.

The advantage of this style is that, the leader has a great deal of control over what's happening. On the other hand, this style has the most negative impact on employees because the coercive style is inflexible, provides little reward. This style should only be used for a short period of time. Avoid excessive use of coercive power.

Transactional – Also known as managerial leadership, the leader focuses on the accomplishment of tasks and good work relationships. In this style, leaders use rewards when performance meets or exceeds expectations and punishment when performance is below expectations. One of the benefits of this style is its simplicity, as rewards and punishments are easily understood by all. This style is required when the leader wants to be in control and when there are approaching deadlines that must be met. Short term goals are achieved quickly with this leadership style. Rewards are powerful motivators but the inspirational effects of rewards are short term. However, in this style since the team runs behind performance and deadlines so there will be fewer chances of innovation and creativity.

Transformational – Transformation is about turning aspirations into reality and converting setbacks into opportunities. This style transforms people as it is associated with change, innovation and entrepreneurship. The objective of this style is to 'transform' people's thinking so that they want to work toward improving the organization and taking it to the next level. Leaders not only concerned and involved in the process, but also focused on helping the team succeed as well. This style assumes that people will follow a person who inspires them. Transformational leaders instil feelings of confidence, admiration and commitment in the team members. Today, organisations need transformational leaders who can convert the organisation into a world-class one.

One of the best uses of this leadership style is in an organisation that is obsolete and requires serious renovation. This style is required when leaders want members to be an active part of the organisation and have ownership to it. Transformational leadership style is more strongly correlated with higher productivity, and higher employee satisfaction.

Since leadership is a complicated issue, hence there is no single correct management leadership style. 'And often the best leaders combine different methods, changing up their styles as the situation changes.' Understanding your leadership style can increase your effectiveness.

SITUATIONAL LEADERSHIP

Leadership is an influential process. When you are a leader, you work with medical representatives to help them accomplish their goals and the goals of the organisation. Leaders are always challenged differently in various situations. The Situational Leadership Model recommends that there is no "one size fits all" approach to leadership. Situational leadership is an adaptive leadership style. This style encourages leaders to choose the leadership style that best fits their goals and circumstances.

> ***There is no best leadership style; it depends on situation and the best leaders are situational.***

The distinction between situational leadership and other leadership styles is that situational leadership incorporates many different techniques. This style relies on Company's environment and the skills and commitment of its followers.

The **Situational Leadership Model** developed by Dr. Paul Hersey and Blanchard in the late 1960s. This model was first called the *'Life Cycle Theory of Leadership.'* During the mid-1970s, it was renamed the situational leadership theory. The **Situational Leadership Model** is very powerful, yet flexible tool that enables first-line leaders to more effectively influence medical representatives. This model states that in modern world, a leader cannot just depend on one management style to fit all situations. Leaders must be flexible in their styles, in order to get the best out of their teams. *'In Situational leadership models, leaders place more or less emphasis on the task, and more or less emphasis on the empowerment of the people they are leading, depending on what's needed to get the job done successfully.'*

> ***'Situational leadership often called organised common sense.'***

The model basically says that the leadership method one employs depends on the situation. First, the leader must identify their most important tasks or priorities. Second, the leader must consider the preparation level of their team members by analysing their ability and willingness. Depending on the level of these variables, leaders must apply the most suitable leadership style to fit the given situation.

Situational Leadership is a combination of directive and supportive behaviours. **Directive behaviour** is characterised as telling, and showing team members what, when and how to do it. **Supportive behaviour** involves praising, listening, encouraging team members in decision-making.

In our context, Situational Leadership style is based on the amount of directive and supportive behaviour given to medical representatives by their first-line leaders. There are four leadership styles comprising of four different mixes of Directive and Supportive Behaviours –

- Directing
- Coaching
- Supporting
- Delegating

There are three steps of the Situational Leadership Model. These are –

Step 1: Identify your most important tasks.

Step 2: Diagnose the readiness level of the medical representatives.

Step 3: Decide the matching leadership style.

Leadership Styles

Supportive Behaviour (Low → High)	Low Directive	High Directive
High	***SUPPORTING*** High Supportive Low Directive	***COACHING*** High Supportive High Directive
Low	***DELEGATING*** Low Supportive Low	***DIRECTING*** Low Supportive High Directive

Low → High
Directive Behaviour

Directing – This leadership approach is most suitable when the medical representatives have low willingness and low ability for the tasks at hand. At the point when the medical representatives cannot do the job and are unwilling or hesitant to attempt, then the first-line leader must take a highly directive role. Directing requires those in charge to define the roles and tasks of the medical representatives, and supervise them closely.

Coaching – This leadership approach is most suitable when the medical representatives have high willingness but low ability for the task at hand. Like directing, coaching still requires first-line leaders to define roles and tasks clearly, and also seeks ideas and recommendations from the medical representatives. While coaching, the first-line leader spends time in listening, advising, and helping the medical representatives gain necessary skills in order to do the task autonomously next time.

Supporting – This leadership approach is most suitable when the medical representatives have low willingness but high ability for the task at hand. Supportive leadership works when the medical representatives can do the job, but is refusing to do it or showing a lack of commitment. Here you need not stress over demonstrating to them what to do, but instead should be concerned with finding out why the medical representative is refusing and work to persuade them to cooperate. The key to supportive leadership is motivating and building confidence in medical representatives. Supportive leadership involves listening, giving praise and making the medical representatives feel good when they show the necessary commitments for success.

Delegating – This leadership approach is most appropriate when the medical representatives have high willingness and high ability. You should rely on delegating when the medical representative can do the job and is motivated to do it. There is a high amount of trust that the medical representatives will do well, and requires little supervision or support. Delegating still keeps the leader involved in the decisions and problem-solving, but execution is mostly in the hands of the medical representatives. Delegation is good management and a sign of strength.

Team Effectiveness – When your team is well established and performs well, you are more likely to apply supporting or delegation styles, because your team members are ready for this. On the other hand, for new teams, or when you take control of an existing team for the first time you will have to utilise the Directing style initially as you must establish yourself among the team and make them work to a high level. This requires high levels of direction and control at the initial stages. After some time, as the team develops in the way that you want, you would then be able to move towards supporting or delegation styles.

Situational Leadership focuses on flexibility and simplicity in execution. This model prepares leaders to address the most urgent challenges that affect in today's work environment. There are three skills of a situational leader –

1. **Diagnosis** – The willingness and ability to look at a situation and assess other's development needs in order to decide which leadership style is the most important for the goal or task at hand.
2. **Flexibility** – The ability to use a variety of leadership styles comfortably. This can be illustrated by the following:

   'Think about driving your car. What would it be like if you could only drive your car in one gear? Just like it is useful to be able to use all the gears (including reverse) in driving a car, it is important to be able to use all of the leadership styles when influencing others. It's important to be more of an all-terrain vehicle, this means flexibility.'

3. **Partnering** – Leadership is a partnership. By making leadership more of a partnership, medical representatives will give first-line leaders the right to lead when they think their leaders have the expertise to help them achieve individual and organisational goals. Partnering is about how to work together effectively with medical representatives to develop their competence and commitment.

> ***'In the past leader was a boss. Today's leader must be partner with people...they no longer can lead solely based on positional power.'***
>
> ***– Ken Blanchard***

Diagnosing Development Level

Development level is task specific. There are two aspects to development level, which first-line leaders should develop for their medical representatives to be self-motivated rather than dependent.

1. Competence
2. Commitment

You have to develop the competence and commitment of your medical representatives so that they become self-motivated rather than dependent on others for direction and guidance. According to Ken Blanchard, *'Four combinations of competence and commitment make up what we call development level.'*

There are four development levels:

- **D1** – Low competence and high commitment
- **D2** – Low competence and low commitment
- **D3** – High competence and low/variable commitment
- **D4** – High competence and high commitment

D4	D3	D2	D1
High Competence High Commitment	High Competence Variable Commitment	Low/some Competence Low Commitment	Low Competence High Commitment
Developed ←			Developing

D1: This level is characterised by a low level of competence and yet, a high level of commitment. This situation is typically with newly joined medical representatives, but sometimes senior medical representatives with new tasks or jobs. At this level, medical representatives are interested in and enthusiastic about the goals or task. They are very eager to learn; willing to take direction. This level requires a leadership style of **Directing** (S1).

D2: At this level the medical representatives have gained some competence or skills, but they lack commitment particularly if the job didn't add up to what they thought it should be. They are discouraged, overwhelmed and confused. **Coaching** (S2) is the actual style of leadership for this level.

D3: The medical representatives at this level have a high level of competence (they know the work); but variable commitment to the job which can affect motivation. Here medical representatives have roadblocks that are preventing them from having a consistent high level of commitment to the job. The style best for this development level is **Supporting** (S3).

D4: The medical representatives at this level are your star performers; they have a high level of both competence and commitment. They are ready to take on new challenges, work independently. They should be led with leadership style **Delegating** (S4).

> ***Leadership style must match the development level. Situational Leadership is not something you do 'TO' people but something you do 'WITH' the people.***

First-line leader and Situational Leadership

- First-line leaders must adapt situational leadership models in every situation as success relies on the flexibility of the approach.
- Medical representatives are not homogenous when it comes to competency and commitment. This model helps leaders to understand the correct way to guide and motivate their medical representatives.
- This model can help first-line leaders to improve their diagnosis and awareness level.
- By understanding the needs of medical representatives, as well as the demands of the task, you can show more empathy, efficiency and flexibility, which can help boost team morale and even enhance productivity.
- The ability to fit one's approach to a specific situation can be strength in today's increasingly changing business environment.

BIBLIOGRAPHY

1. Vivek Hattangadi. "Pharma First Line Leader to CEO," The road map to success. Pothi.com
2. John C. Maxwell. "The 21 Indispensable Qualities of a Leader," Magna Publishing Co. Ltd.
3. John C. Maxwell. "Attitude," Jaico Publishing House.
4. Donald H. Weiss. "Effective Team Building," Goyal Publishers and Distributors Pvt. Ltd.
5. John Adair. "Effective Leadership," Pan Books.
6. John Adair. "Effective Motivation," Pan Books.
7. John Adair. "Decision-Making and Problem-Solving," Kogan Page.
8. Daniel Golman. "Working With Emotional Intelligence," Bloomsbury.
9. Pramod Batra and Vijay Batra. "Management Thoughts," Full Circle.
10. John Adair. "Develop your leadership skills," Kogan Page.
11. Stephen R. Covey. "The 7 Habits of Highly Effective People," Simon and Schuster.
12. Arati Gaurav. "Time Management," Buzzingstock Publishing House.
13. Arati Gaurav. "Leadership + Teamwork = Success," Buzzingstock Publishing House.
14. Radhakrishnan Pillai and D. Sivanandhan. "Chanakya's 7 Secrets of Leadership," Jaico Publishing House.
15. Allan Pease. "Body Language," Manjul Publishing House.
16. Pramod Batra. "Born To Win," Full Circle Publishing.
17. Napoleon Hill. "Think and Grow Rich," Amazing Reads.
18. Ken Blanchard. "Leadership By The Book," Harper Collins Publishers.
19. Dr. Joseph Murphy. 'Believe in Yourself,' Manjul Publishing House.

20. Ramesh K. Arora. 'Art of Leadership,' Paragon International Publishers.
21. Mitesh Khatri and Indu Khatri. 'Awaken The Leader In You,' Jaico Publishing House.
22. Alison Price and David Price. 'Leadership A practical guide,' Introducingbooks.com
23. Mark Miller. 'The Heart of Leadership,' Berret-Koehler Publishers.
24. Brain Tracy. 'Effective Leadership,' Jaico Publishing House.
25. Meera Johri. 'Inspiring Thoughts on successful Leadership,' Rajpal and Sons.
26. Robin Sarma. "The Leader Who Had No Title," Jaico Publishing House.
27. Robin Sarma. "Leadership Wisdom," Jaico Publishing House.
28. Anup Soans. "Supervision For The Super Wiser Front –Line Manager," Asian Trading Corporation.
29. Leena Sen. "Communication Skills," PHI Learning Pvt. Ltd.
30. Ashish Dutta. "Body Language," Goodwill Publishing House.
31. Peter Simon. "Communication Skills," Reader's Delight.
32. C. Lakshman. "Knowledge Leadership," Response.
33. Prakash Iyer. "The Secret of Leadership," Portfolio Penguin.
34. Dr. Sanjiv Chopra. "Leadership By Example," Thomas Dunne Books.
35. Sue Bishop. "Develop Your Assertiveness," Kogan Page India Pvt. Ltd.
36. Simon Sinek. 'Start With Why,' Portfolio Penguin.
37. Vivek Mehrotra. "Why my horse doesn't drink," Viva books Pvt. Ltd.
38. Vivek Mehrotra. "Why my horse doesn't Listen," Viva books Pvt. Ltd.
39. Vivek Mehrotra. "Essential of Pharmaceutical sales Management," Foundation Books.
40. Keneth Blanchard. 'The one minute manager,' Harper Collins.
41. Cynthia Kersey. 'Unstoppable' Magna Books division.
42. Shiv Khera. 'You can sell,' Rupa Publications.

43. Shiv Khera. 'You can Win,' Macmillan India Ltd.

44. Dale Carnegie. 'The Leader in You,' Sulabh Publications.

45. Dale Carnegie. 'How to Win Friends and Influence People,' Replica Press Pvt. Ltd.

46. Normal Vincent Peale. "The Power of Positive Thinking," Vermilion.

47. William Walker Atkinson. "The Secret of Success," Good Books Distributors Publishers.

48. Vivek Hattangadi. 'Total Communication,' Pothi.com

49. Robert K. Greenleaf. 'Servant Leadership,' Magna Books division.

50. Mahesh Baxi. 'New Age Leadership,' Jaico Publishing House.

51. Uday Kumar Haldar. 'Leadership and Team Building,' Oxford University Press.

52. Vivek Mehrotra. 'Why My Horse Doesn't Smile,' Viva Books.

53. Prem P. Bhalla. '7 Steps To Becoming A Leader,' Goodwill Publishing House.

54. Prem P. Bhalla. '7 Steps To Effective Communication,' Goodwill Publishing House.

55. Prem P. Bhalla. '7 Steps To Effective Time Management,' Goodwill Publishing House.

56. Prem P. Bhalla. '7 Steps To Effective Team Building,' Goodwill Publishing House.

57. Dr. Glenn Wilson. 'Body Language,' Icon Books UK.

58. Ken Blanchard and Marc Muchnik. 'The Leadership Pill,' Pocket Books.

59. Arun. H. Raikar. "Discover The Power Within You," Ocean Paperbacks.

60. Jack Trout. "Differentiate or Die," Westland Ltd.

61. Vinay Mohan Sharma. "Gestures & Body Language," V & S Publisher.

62. Geoff Ribbens & Richard Thompson. "Body Language For Management," Hachette India.

63. Brian Tracy. "Sales Management," Manjul Publishing House.

64. Bevoc, Louis. "Leadership Style + Toxic Leadership: 2 Books in 1," NutriNiche System LLC. Kindle Edition.

65. Brian Tracy. "Leadership," Manjul Publishing House Pvt Ltd. Kindle Edition.

66. Gibson Frank. "Leadership." Kindle Edition.

67. Miller Joe. "Body Language," Kindle Edition.

68. Vivek Bindra. "Everything About Leadership." Diamond Pocket Books (P) Ltd. Kindle Edition.

69. Goldberg, Jason. "Sales Management," Kindle Edition.

70. James Linda & Olga Smith. "Pace, Pitch, Pause, Power," BATCS Global. Kindle Edition.

71. Vivek Bindra. "Double Your Growth Through Excellent Customer Service," Diamond Pocket Books (P) Ltd. Kindle Edition.

72. Vivek Bindra. "Effective Planning and Time Management," Bloomsbury Publishing. Kindle Edition.

73. T. V. Rao. "IIMA – Managers Who Make A Difference: Sharpening Your Management Skills," Random House Publishers India Pvt. Ltd. Kindle Edition.

74. Brian Tracy. "Delegation and Supervision." Manjul Publishing House Pvt Ltd. Kindle Edition.